THE COOKIE BOOK

"Reading *The Cookie Book* epitomizes 'sexuality' to me — an experience in which one's senses are simultaneously assaulted, culminating and forever feeling alive, woman, wild and wonderful. Like sexuality, Maritza's book is multi-layered and well researched with mixed medias, from cartoon strips to poetry and gorgeous illustrations, to keep the reader constantly alert, educated and interested. A beautiful contribution to women and their sexuality."
— Dr. Marlene Wasserman, aka Dr. Eve, author, registered sex therapist in South Africa and the USA, lecturer, and radio talk-show host

"What a refreshing and candid look at something we all want to know more about and discuss but often do not! Maritza has managed to educate, make one laugh and be amazed all at the same time, and it's all delivered with such humor, passion and love for her subject. This is a must-read for all the women out there and for any man who likes women and wants to know more!"
— Embeth Davidtz, actress

"Absolutely beautiful and well-written…filled with vital information."
— Nancy Richards, author and radio talk-show host

"From the cultural importance of virginity to how the cookie crumbles as we age and how and why people groom and adorn their 'lovely lady part' this creative little book will educate you on all things vaginal."
— Lesley Byram, *Cape Times*

"Funny and creative with beautiful artworks… celebrates the best of being female."
— Nicole Sparrow, *Longevity Magazine*

"It is a small, beautifully illustrated booklet that certainly packs a punch. When it comes to the health and understanding of one's 'private zones' one simply has to call a spade a spade — and this book does just that."
— *Odyssey Magazine*

"Recognizing the importance and profundity of the vagina… philosophical and humorous… a tome that admirably attempts to unravel and ponder the history, impact and beauty of the vagina."
— Oliver Roberts, *Sunday Times*

"Inspirational, creatively illustrated…delightful… should be given to all teenage girls."
— Vivien Horler, *Cape Argus*

The Cookie Book

Celebrating the Art, Power and Mystery
of Women's Sweetest Spot

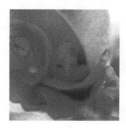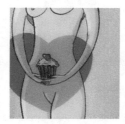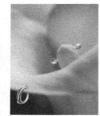

Maritza Breitenbach

Hunter House PUBLISHERS

Hunter House Inc., Publishers
PO Box 2914
Alameda CA 94501-0914

Library of Congress Cataloging-in-Publication Data
Breitenbach, Maritza.
The cookie book : celebrating the art, power and mystery of women's
sweetest spot / Maritza Breitenbach.
p. cm.
ISBN 978-0-89793-606-4 (pbk.)
1. Vagina — Popular works.   2. Women — Health and hygiene — Popular
works.   3. Self-care, Health — Popular works.   I. Title.
RG268.B74 2011
611'.67 — dc23   2011030595

Project Credits

Cover Design: Brian Dittmar Design, Inc.	Special Sales Manager: Judy Hardin
Book Production: John McKercher	Rights Coordinator: Candace Groskreutz
Copy Editor: Amy Bauman	Customer Service Manager: Christina Sverdrup
Proofreader: Erica M. Lee	Order Fulfillment: Washul Lakdhon
Managing Editor: Alexandra Mummery	Administrator: Theresa Nelson
Acquisitions Assistant: Elana Fiske	Computer Support: Peter Eichelberger
Publisher: Kiran S. Rana	

9 8 7 6 5 4 3 2   First Edition   12 13 14 15 16

CONTENTS

LIST OF IMAGES

DEDICATION

To the memory of Jacqueline Breitenbach

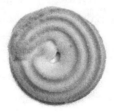

PREFACE

"Why a book about the vagina?" I often asked myself when I'd wake up in the middle of the night. Why would *anyone,* other than a medical specialist or a pornographer, attempt to breach such a taboo subject? To answer this question I first need to explain how this book came into being.

I have always taken pride in enjoying open and easy communication with my children. That was until one Sunday afternoon when my daughter needed some advice on intimate care and hygiene. I was baffled, uncomfortable, embarrassed, and caught off guard. I lacked the knowledge and correct vocabulary to answer a very simple question. This scenario made me realize that issues surrounding the female genitalia are shrouded in secrecy and that general, but vital, information is often scarce and scattered. I had to learn more.

I started having conversations with other women of all ages. Apart from having loads of fun and laughter, it saddened me to realize that these get-togethers often offered the first platform for members of the fairer sex to discuss problems, share experiences, and gain information about this small, yet powerful, aspect of our being. It came as no surprise to find that we all needed advice about our intimate bits. Most of us had little knowledge of our genital anatomy; we were deficient in the correct vocabulary and were unsure about what is and is not considered "normal." Some women have never even taken a glimpse at their own vaginas, and those who had were often concerned about what they discovered. The younger crowd had questions about the hymen and sexual intercourse, as well as other, more delicate matters; mothers were concerned about not having enough information and confidence to guide their daughters through puberty into womanhood. Some ladies were overwhelmed by menopausal changes and had many questions that were not serious enough to take to a medical practitioner but still needed answering. The questions and concerns were endless—it was clearly a topic that had been neglected for far too long.

Armed with a master's degree in biomedical ethics, a great love for research, and a deep-seated dedication to the project, I endeavored to gather useful information and reintroduce the topic in a format that is easily digestible and a pleasure to read. Endless hours of research led me on the most enlightening journey of discovery—the information I found, often hidden deeply in medical journals and research papers, was both valuable and fascinating.

I envisioned an informal book that would resonate with all women and their loved ones, a book that does not contain too much detailed or specialized information but still manages to answers all the niggling questions we often have but are too embarrassed to talk about. Furthermore, I intended to create a work filled with beautiful graphics, illustrations, and photographs that plays on the lighter side of things but also reflects the delicate and complex nature of this exquisite little organ, the vagina.

I am extremely blessed that this book has managed to achieve just that. It certainly has been a daunting task, and I had to muster all my courage and incur a fair amount of criticism in realizing this book. Even my teenage son wanted to disown me, and he cringed with embarrassment until his male friends caught wind of the topic and started asking questions of their own. Only then, after they approved, did it become more acceptable to him, even "cool."

I sincerely hope that you will find as much personal value and enlightenment in this book as I have had in writing it. May it always remind you of the mirth, magic, and mystery of your sweetest spot. May it transport you on a journey of discovery as it accompanies you and yours on the lifecycle from infancy to puberty, from sexual maturity to giving birth, menopause, and beyond. May it instill pride in you and give you a confident voice, strengthened with all the knowledge you need to take care of, understand, embrace, and celebrate your unique womanness.

ACKNOWLEDGMENTS

I wish to express my sincere thanks and appreciation to all of those who made this journey possible.

First of all, I am eternally grateful for Hunter House Publishers, USA, who granted me the honor and privilege of being published internationally. My heartfelt thanks to the whole team but more specifically to the following individuals: Kiran Rana, who is responsible for giving this book a chance and whose constant support and wonderfully insightful comments and suggestions have been instrumental in helping me polish the final product. Elizabeth Kracht, Alex Mummery, and her team, Amy Bauman and Erica M. Lee, for their intense attention to the grammar, punctuation, and spelling. John McKercher for his meticulous attention to the final book design and layout.

Furthermore, I wish to express my appreciation to the medical professionals, sexologists, scientists, reporters, authors, and academics across the centuries who provided all of the facts contained in this book. It has been a tremendous privilege to gain knowledge and understanding from their work. With admiration for their unflagging dedication to women's health issues, I salute them. Special thanks to Dr. Cathy Agnew from the Women's Wellness Clinic in Somerset West, who double-checked the medical information. It is, however, possible that I have made errors in the interpretation of these facts, and for any errors I take full responsibility.

My gratitude goes to my local team from the city of Cape Town, South Africa, who supported, challenged, and cheered: Minette Goosen, the "cookie cutter" from In Touch Skincare and Nail Studio, who skillfully plucked, bleached, styled, and colored our models' pubic hair. Our models: These brave women good-humoredly endured the pain of pubic grooming and henna tattooing and then flounced for the camera. Milan Cronje, a well-known international fashion photographer, was responsible for taking the "drop shots"—he effortlessly put our models at ease and created beautiful photographic artworks.

A huge thank you goes to Italian-born Filippo ioco (sic), world-renowned body-painting artist, who generously provided me with the images of his magnificent creations. I also applaud Ronelle van Zyl from Graffic Traffic, Cape Town, South Africa, who, with equanimity and ingenuity, prepared the graphics for the book.

Then there are "my own people," who often lost me to the task of exploring this subject: Sylvia Niewergeldt, who supplied endless cups of fresh coffee while taking care of the household chores; the man in my life who initiated the idea of this book, and my three wonderful children. Without the miracle of these individuals, I could not have embarked on this venture; they have been patient, supportive, and loving, as always. I shall also be eternally grateful to my late parents who influenced my thinking enormously—especially my mother, who's endearing and mischievous nature has been a source of inspiration to me.

Lastly and most of all I would like to acknowledge you, the reader. Contained in this book I believe is vital information that I hope will be of tremendous benefit. I applaud you for your insight and courage. Enjoy, and please recommend this book or pass it on to all whom you feel may benefit from the content: Knowing more about women's sweetest spot is indeed a powerful delight!

IMPORTANT NOTE

The material in this book is intended to provide a review of information regarding female sexuality. Every effort has been made to provide accurate and dependable information. We believe any advice given in this book poses no risk to any healthy person. However, if you have any recurring problems, or suspect that you may be suffering from a sexually transmitted disease, we strongly recommend consulting your doctor.

The publisher, authors, and editors, as well as the professionals quoted in the book, cannot be held responsible for any error, omission, professional disagreement, or dated material, and are not liable for any damage, injury, or other adverse outcome of applying any of the information resources in this book. If you have questions concerning the application of the information described in this book, consult a qualified professional.

What could be better than our nicely tapered entrance?

It's discreet and stylish, everything is cleverly and compactly encased in

the body … there's a neat triangle of hair above it,

like a road sign, should you lose your way — it's perfect.

— Yann Martel, *Self*

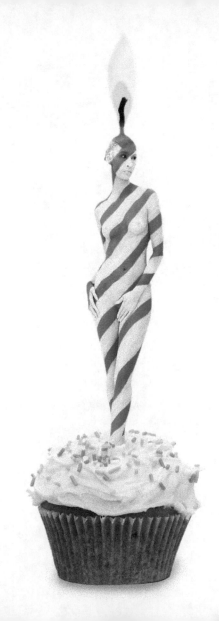

Filippo ioco, *Birthday Girl*

INTRODUCTION

Is the vagina a fleshy fruit (a mango or an apricot), fragrant treat (a muffin or a pie), or something sweet (fudge, a cookie, a jam donut), or is it something dangerous like the Bermuda triangle or a squirrel trap? Better yet, is it an animal (a beaver, a pussycat, a monkey, or a rat), a container of sorts (a Pandora's Box, a cubbyhole, a honey pot), or a childishly or nonsensically named body part (hoo-hoo, choo-choo or nuki-tuki)? Is "she" a person in her own right (Betty, Fanny, Nan)? Is it the highway to heaven or simply "downstairs"; or is it a natural phenomenon (a cave, a bush, a flower, a jungle, a forest)?

The vagina has been showered with terms such as "life-affirming," "iconic," "mystical," and "divine." Throughout history it has been said that once exposed, the vagina possesses the power to frighten gods, to drive out evil spirits, or to promote harvest fertility. A Catalan saying, *"La mar es posa bona si veu el cony d'una dona,"* tells us that the sea calms down if it sees a woman's vagina, yet some of us have never even caught a glimpse of our own.

Let's not beat around the bush any longer. Brace yourself and join me as we explore and celebrate these secret, fleshy folds we call our own.

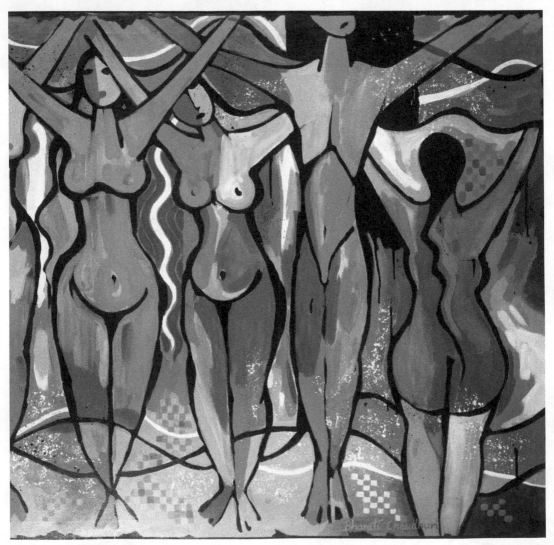

Bharati Chaudhuri, *Freedom*

PART I

UNVEILING THE
WOMEN'S SECRET

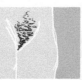
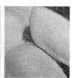

CHAPTER 1

NAMING OUR SOFT SPOT

During this exploratory journey, I found two sad-but-truisms. The first: Often when the subject in question is mentioned, some people gasp in embarrassment, others giggle, eyes shy away, and facial expressions convey anything from surprise to disapproval to complete shock. The second: Most of us seem to struggle to find a name for our lovely lady parts. In our quest to find a name, we lean heavily on euphemisms such as "down there" as substitute expressions. The phrase "women's secret" was the collective generic term used during the Middle Ages, and in this typical endeavor to obscure the subject in question, Sigmund Freud called it "the dark continent." Apparently we are still very much in the dark, as the mystery surrounding female sexuality is clearly reflected in the scarcity of appropriate words.

In colloquial speech, the term *vagina* is commonly but incorrectly used to refer to the female genitalia. Strictly speaking, the vagina is a specific internal structure, whereas the *vulva*, in reality, refers to the exterior genitalia. Noticeably, hardly any woman talks about her vulva when referring to that special place, and seemingly we are not that comfortable with the term *vagina* either. Vagina sounds almost too clinical and seems to work best in conversations between doctor and patient as it is most often used in medical jargon. And since most of us are a little confused about what exactly the *labia majora, labia minora, mons pubis, clitoris, greater and lesser vestibular glands, and vaginal orifice* refer to, we comfortably get away with calling them all "private parts."

According to Steven Pinker, a psychology professor at Harvard and the author of *The Stuff of Thought: Language as a Window into Human Nature*, at least 1,200 terms have been used for the vagina throughout the history of the English language. Among the array of possibilities, we find some silly but arguably cute names such as *fanny, cookie, thingy, pundge, tukie, nuki, cooter, coochie, punani, vadge, hey nonny nonny, hot cha-cha, honey pot, Lady Jane, yum-yum,* and *vajayjay.* Yoni, a Sanskrit word with positive and sacred undertones, meaning "the source of life" and "divine passage," is gaining ground in the effort to find an appropriate term.

Expressions of a more vulgar variety, often favored by young men, are *beaver, bush, camel-toe* (the outline of the vagina when made visible through tight-fitting pants), *mango-pip, apricot split, quack, gwarr, slit,* and *crack.* There are, of course, other names with which we are familiar. Perhaps we have heard these words when insults are thrown around in a crude and demeaning manner, or we may have seen them as graffiti inscribed on the odd public toilet door or when used in steamy pornography and erotica. Unfortunately these words, and the way in which they're often used, add to the distorted perspective many women have about their vaginas. Instead of promoting a healthy body image, these expressions strengthen the hypersexualized and shame-based views that we hold.

One could draw naming ideas from related words, such as the *perineal sponge* (the pad between the vagina and the rectum), and call our most intimate parts our *periwinkle,* but then

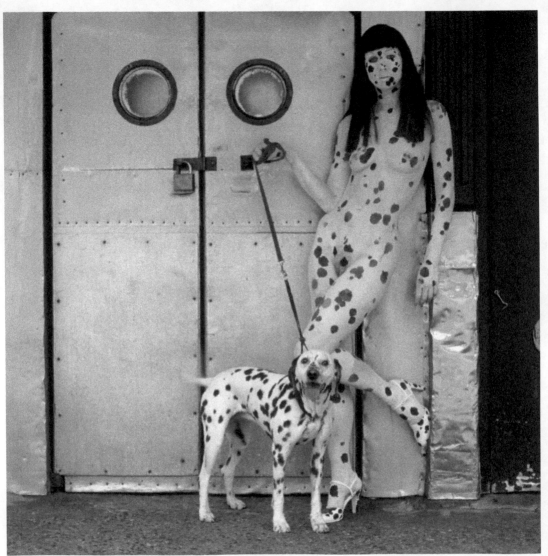

Filippo ioco, *Walk Me*

again, it is neither a pale, bluish purple flower, nor is it an edible sea snail. The fact remains that our most secret and treasured body part goes by the uncompromisingly clinical term *va-jine-na,* and even after discovering the exquisiteness and wonder surrounding the subject, we find this term blunt, unappealing, and downright dreadful. Words like *belly button*, *tummy, eyes,* and *toes* flow softly off the tongue, but *vagina* or *vulva!* I rest my case.

Calling our vaginas by any other name is not necessarily derogatory; there is a place for pet names that can be used in a familiar and playful manner among friends and family. On the other hand, Eve Ensler, a prominent antiviolence activist, playwright, and creator of *The Vagina Monologues,* warns that "what we don't say becomes a secret, and secrets often create shame and fear and myths." If this is the case, it is perhaps time for us to get off the euphemism treadmill.

VAGINA, THE TRAVELER'S GUIDE	
Afrikaans	vagina
Albanian	vaginë
Czech	pochva, vagína
Dutch	vagina, schede, kut
Estonian	vagiina, tupp
Filipino	kaluban, puki
Finnish	vagina, emätin
French	vagin, barbu, bonbonnière
Galician	vaxina
German	vagina, scheide, schoß, kut
Greek	moonie, konnos, kunthus
Hungarian	vagina, hüvely
Indonesian	farji, puki, pukas, vagina
Italian	vagina
Latin	pudenda, concha
Polish	pochwa
Portuguese	vagina
Spanish	vagina
Swedish	vagina, sköte, slida
Turkish	vajina, dölyolu
Vietnamese	âm đạo
Yiddish	vagine, lock hole, k'nish

CHAPTER 2

BY THE LOOKS OF THINGS

Every woman is a mystery to be solved. But truth be told, one is taken aback and left somewhat bewildered and speechless after using a mirror for the first time to inspect one's own "dark continent." Although mystifying, it does somewhat look like an injury or, at least, like an untidy, unlovely design. However, once we get to know this unique and wondrous component of our being, it will leave us feeling liberated and, ultimately, feminine.

At the upper, exterior tip of the boat-shaped vulva lies the *mons veneris* (also known as the *pubic mound,* the *Mound of Venus*, the *mons pubis*, or simply the *mons)* and just beneath it, in the upper folds of the *labia* ("lips"), we find the *clitoris* neatly hidden under a thick fold of skin. This female sexual organ, revealing itself like a little button, is found in all female mammals — with the exception of the spotted hyena, which has a fully erectile pseudo-penis that is used for urination, mating, and giving birth.

Since this small, exquisitely sensitive organ is exclusively there to tickle our fancy, it merits our special attention. The word *clitoris* derives from the Greek word *kleitorid,* which literally means "little hill," but this is just the tip of the iceberg!

Recent studies have proven that the clitoris is, in fact, much larger than we ever imagined. Although the visible part (the clitoral gland) is pealike in size, it, in actual fact, extends into the vaginal wall: According to Williamson and Nowak, "[t]he 'body' of the clitoris, which connects to the glans, is about as big as the first joint of your thumb. It

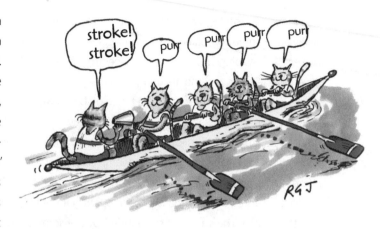

has two arms of up to 9 centimeters [4 inches] long (!) that flare backwards into the body, lying just a few millimeters from the ends of the muscles that run up the inside of the thigh."

During sex, this entire structure, which is wrapped around the urethra and the vagina, becomes engorged. And it has the most explosive qualities: During stimulation, the visible clitoral gland, which is densely packed with as many as eight thousand nerve endings, puffs out and changes color as the erectile tissue fills with blood. Isn't it delightful to know that our pleasure button is not just an abbreviation of sorts, but that its wonderful, tantalizing qualities actually spread into all the nooks and crannies of our fannies? Why our sex organ has been condensed so drastically is a mystery, but at least now we have the whole clitoral truth.

Let's paddle farther up the creek: The hair-covered, outer lips extending from the mons veneris are called the *labia majora*. They are irregular in shape and thick and fleshy, and not nearly as neat and tidy as one would have hoped. In terms of hues, we are looking at combinations and variations of tawny or dark brown, coffee, plum, slate gray, and black. The rosy inner lips, the *labia minora,* appear to curve out and over the outer labia. These are quite fleshy and can be compared to the softly curled and intricate petal shapes that we find in exotic flowers such as orchids. Here the color spectrum includes shades of violet, lavender, and indigo; covering the pinks, we find anything from dusky to cherry to crimson to salmon; in a bluish tint we may discover raspberry, and for a touch of "bling," we even have golden ochre! During sexual arousal and pregnancy, these colors deepen a little and, since the lips puff out, they appear even more spectacular; after childbirth the colors become more blue, and after menopause shades become a softer, rosy gray. Like colors on a canvas, or like musical tones, it is an extraordinary *chef d'œuvre,* a matchless masterpiece. Don't you think?

Neatly tucked away in the middle of our frilly inner lips, we find the opening of the urethra and the vagina. The vagina is surrounded by pelvic muscles that form a figure eight around both the vagina and the anus; these can be felt if we insert our fingers inside our vaginas and squeeze. These muscles, which contract at 0.8-second intervals during orgasms, are rich in nerve endings that record and increase pleasurable sensations to enhance our sexual adventures. It is most important to exercise these muscles on a regular basis since strong pelvic muscles not only strengthen the *pubococcygeus (PC)* muscles (the muscles that run between the vagina and the anus, sometimes referred to as "the hooch," I hear), but they also prevent and control burdensome urinary incontinence (the "laugh-and-leak" effect) and pelvic organ prolapse. These exercises are known as Kegel exercises, and although most of us don't jump for joy at the prospect of a workout in any shape or form, this foray into exercise, once a regular practice, guarantees many lasting benefits.

Here goes:

- Empty your bladder and sit or lie down.
- Contract your pelvic floor muscles.

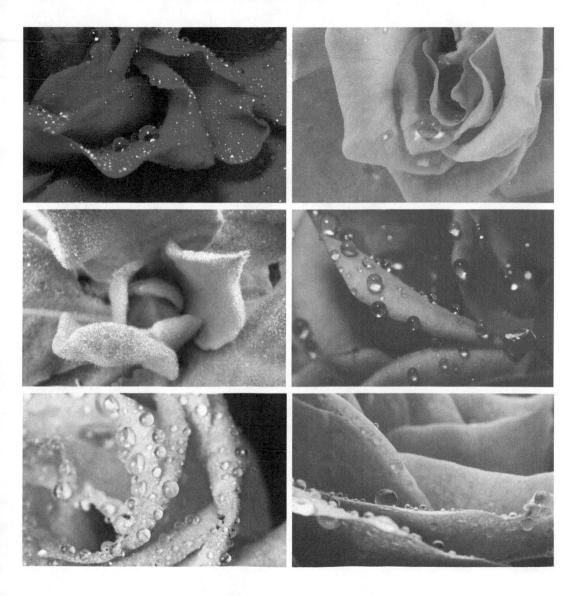

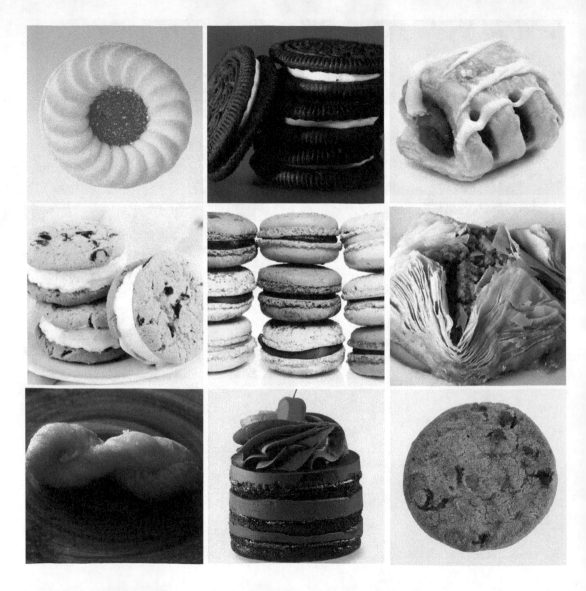

- Be careful not to flex the muscles in your abdomen, thighs, or buttocks.

- Relax, breathe freely, and focus on tightening the muscles around your vagina and rectum.

- Hold for three seconds and then relax for three seconds.

- Repeat ten times.

- Work up to keeping the muscle contractions for ten seconds at a time, relaxing for ten seconds between contractions.

Now that we have flexed our muscles, like any tough cookie should, and examined the ins and outs of our vaginas, little remains to be said about the basic anatomy but this: Every nook and cranny of our vaginas is perfectly imperfect—our own unique, private Eden. So whether you're the owner of a petite *fortune-cookie,* a *macaroon*, a *snickerdoodle*, or a *chocolate brownie*, learn to live with it, and love it shamelessly!

THE JOY OF THE G-SPOT: FACT OR FALLACY?

In 1950, Dr. Ernst Gräfenberg, a German gynecologist, surmised that the anterior wall of the vagina along the urethra is the seat of a distinct erogenous zone. The term "G-spot," which is an abbreviation for the Gräfenberg Spot, wasn't coined until much later, in a case study on female ejaculation. Based on these findings, *The G-Spot and Other Recent Discoveries about Human Sexuality* was published the following year. Curiosity about the discovery of this erogenous patch was piqued: The book became a best-seller overnight and consequently was translated into nineteen languages.

The G-spot remains to be a highly controversial topic that is still referred to as a "modern gynecological myth." In a recent comprehensive study of 1,804 British female twins, the authors found no physiological or physical evidence for the presence of the G-spot and argued that the idea of this spot is purely subjective. Rebecca Chalker, the author of *The Clitoral Truth: The Secret World at Your Fingertips*, on the other hand, states that *all* women have a urethral sponge (which can be felt through the vaginal wall) that serves as the G-spot. Deborah Sundahl, author of *Female Ejaculation & the G-Spot*, goes even further: She argues that although the size, shape and amount of pleasure or discomfort we experience during stimulation of the G-spot may vary, that it is quite visible, and that every women's spot can, in fact, be seen.

Other researchers claim that the G-spot does exist but that not all women appear to have one, and that among those who do, 82 percent of women report vaginal orgasms and approximately 10 percent experience ejaculation. This view is supported by the findings of an Italian medical team from the University of L'Aquila, Italy, who reported they had performed ultrasound scans on twenty women and that about half of them had a "thickened area" between the vagina and the urethra. Saeed Mohamad Ahmad Thaber similarly found in a study of 175 women from Cairo that the G-spot is a functional reality in 82.3 percent of women, an anatomical reality in 54.3 percent of women, and a histological reality in 47.4 percent of women (a "functional reality" refers to women's own perception of hightened sensation, an "anatomical reality" indicates physical evidence, and a "histological reality" refers to the microscopic proof of cell and tissue matter).

Another fascinating research study shows that stimulation of the G-spot area raises the pain threshold of a woman by 47 percent. If the stimulus is continued until arousal occurs, the pain threshold increases by 84 percent, followed by a massive 107 percent when we indulge ourselves in orgasmic delight. These findings suggest that this sensitive area serves as a natural painkiller that is helpful during childbirth.

Although researchers are still at loggerheads about the existence of the elusive G-spot, this is no reason to abandon the idea just yet. Let us see if *we* can hit the spot....

This region is said to be of thicker and slightly coarser tissue, with a texture similar to that of a walnut. It is located 1 to 2 inches from the opening of the vagina on the front wall, and it can be stimulated with a "come-here" movement of the index or middle finger. Now is a good time to solicit the assistance of your partner, who will surely be delighted to accompany you on this journey of discovery. First and foremost, it is best to be sexually aroused before we venture to this spongy area, which will be engorged by the excitement phase. In the pre-excitement stage, this area is no bigger than a pea, but once aroused, it doubles in size (or grows even bigger than that). Have your partner gently stroke the spot while varying the amount of pressure applied. Some women experience an overwhelming urge to urinate during the stimulation of this area, so make sure your bladder is empty before adding G-spot exploration to your bedroom repertoire.

Your happy hunting will permit you to determine if the G-spot is indeed a fabulously thrilling find or just a misleading fallacy. Perhaps this is another intimate marvel to explore and share? You be the judge....

NIP AND TUCK

Some women find it unacceptable if the labia minora (the small inner folds that surround the openings to the urethra and vagina) protrude past the labia majora (the two large, outer fleshy folds). These women are drawn to a procedure called vaginal labiaplasty. The surgery takes

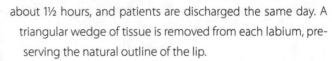

about 1½ hours, and patients are discharged the same day. A triangular wedge of tissue is removed from each labium, preserving the natural outline of the lip.

After the swelling and bruising subside and all the stitches have dissolved, the patient is left with a tiny, horizontal scar on each labium. Apart from some antibiotic gel that needs to be applied for a few days, no special postoperative care is required. Abstinence from sexual activity for six weeks after the procedure is advised to allow the tissues adequate time to heal completely.

Doctors who advocate this procedure claim that women can regain a "youthful look" and guarantee that there will be no disturbance of sensation as a result of this operation. However, my question is this: What is a "youthful look," in this case?

Some young, sexually inexperienced women are naturally endowed with lovely full and fleshy, "mature"-looking genitalia: Does this imply that they are not "youthful" looking? By the same token, we find that some much older and sexually seasoned women's genitalia naturally appear neat and streamlined; are they, therefore, "youthful" *and* mature? It seems like "looking youthful" is merely an interpretation of the wonderful variety that our unique looks offer, and this is incidentally not determined by age or "youthfulness" as such.

As far as vaginal labiaplasty goes, I'd be terrified that too many cooks would spoil my broth, so I'll learn to love my perfectly imperfect design, thank you very much.

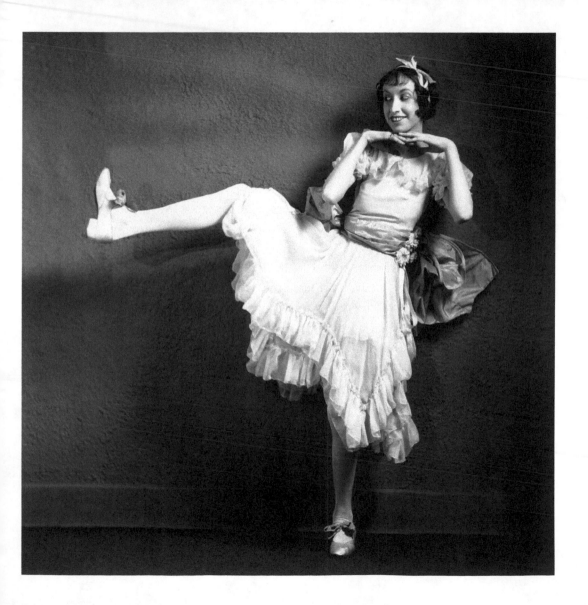

CHAPTER 3

SCENT OF A WOMAN

Vaginal aroma (or *cassolette,* which is French for "perfume or incense burner") is a conversational topic one would certainly not initiate at the dinner table, or any other public gathering for that matter. It goes beyond the pale of subjects that are considered mentionable and is definitely a social taboo. In literature, we observe that many men actually desire a woman's unique *cassolette.* Possibly one of the more celebrated opinions is that of the great emperor of the French, Napoleon Bonaparte (1769–1821), whose preference and rapture for the natural and unwashed smell of his wife, Empress Josephine, are well recorded and rather remarkable. It is said that upon returning home from the battlefield he would send word to Josephine with precise instructions: *"Ne te laves pas, je reviens"* — "Don't wash; I'm coming home." In one of the many love letters he wrote to his wife, one particular sentence stands out and leaves us breathless:

I send a thousand kisses to your neck, your breasts,
and lower down, much lower down, that little black forest I love so well.

We, on the other hand, are decidedly more hesitant about the matter and easily become typical shrinking violets. We take to cowering in the presence of our gynecologist or lover when we feel our scent is somewhat less than rosy even after washing once, twice, and sometimes three times, just for good measure. We are also continually bombarded by advertising and consumer products that encourage us to spray away our natural scent in favor of a more pleasant peaches-and-petals fragrance. After all, we have been told that our perfume, of the kind found in bottles, reveals more about us than our handwriting. It is near impossible to ignore such statements, especially when they come from esteemed fashion royalty such as Christian Dior, who was famously quoted as saying his dream is to "save women from nature"! And then, of course, there are also those dreadful "fishy" jokes, which only add to women's already-lengthy list of insecurities.

Perhaps the notion of deodorizing creates no more than an illusion since some perfumes are, in fact, based on intimate and animal scents that are meant to "awaken bestial cravings in the hygiene-obsessed." Consider this list of French perfumes, for example, which plays on the scent of coitus or sexual intercourse: *Lover* by Editions du Parfum; *Putain des Palaces* (Whore of the Palaces) and *Sécrétions Magnifiques* (Magnificent Secretions) by Etat Libre d'Orange; Alan Cumming's *Cumming;* and Guerlain's *Les Elixirs Charnels* (Carnal Elixers).

Kilian Hennessy describes his perfume, *Liaisons Dangereuses*, as being based on the pleasures that a Parisian orgy offers: "Bodies

Filippo ioco, *Double Scoop*

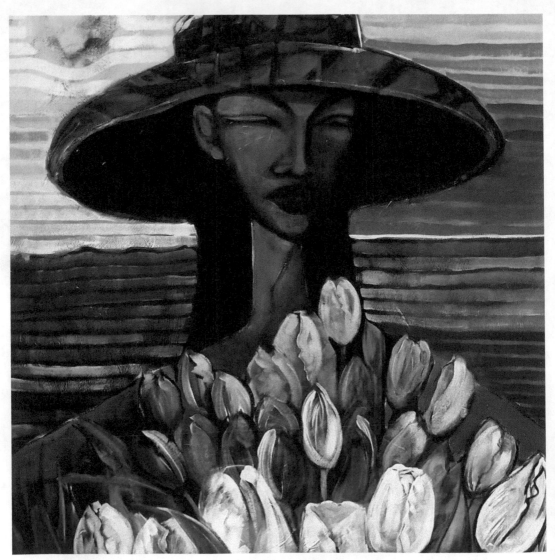

Marsha Hatcher, *Tulip Lady* (2005)

slick with sweat, hot with the odors of sexual favors bestowed and received during the night." *Querelle* by Parfumerie Generale embodies the theme of the Jean Genet novel, *Querelle de Brest* (1947), which focuses on a handsome but immoral sailor who is embroiled in a plot drenched with sexual promiscuity. The French perfumer, Jacques Guerlain (1874–1963) believed that perfume should smell like the underside of his mistress; hence, from the House of Guerlain we discover that both *Jicky* (1889) and *Shalimar* (1925) are tinged with vaginal and anal smells.

The classic way to make French perfume is to include animal scents like musk, castoreum, and ambergris in base notes as fixatives. Musk, which means "testicle" in Sanskrit, fashions an aroma of sweet blood and is derived from the anal gland of the male musk deer and civet cats; castoreum is found in the dried and ground gland pouch of the beaver and adds a leathery tincture to perfumes; ambergris or "amber" is a solid, waxy, dull gray or blackish secretion produced in the digestive system of sperm whales, and it produces a sweet, earthy odor. Based on these key ingredients, we find that *Cruel Intentions* by Kilian smells of leather, urine, smoky tar and anus; Christian Dior's *Dioressence* of fecal notes; *Miss Dior*, which is one of my all-time favorites, like sweaty armpits; and *Black Orchid* by Tom Ford like a man's crotch. Wow!

Another interesting morsel of information — not for the-faint-of-heart but perhaps for the lonesome, companionless consumer — is that you can purchase a tiny glass vial brimming with vaginal fluid from a vendor in Germany. This most intimate of scents is said to drive men absolutely wild, which really shouldn't come as much of a surprise since so many people believe that the *cassolette* of a woman is a sexual treasure to be cherished and revered, a true asset, an inner gem on par with our outer beauty.

These sensual, subtle smells of the body send strong signals to the brain and have the power to tantalize, arouse, and even tickle the taste buds. Whether these responses are based on "pleasure memory" or pheromones (an airborne, odorless chemical signal that triggers a natural response in another member of the same species) is still unclear. For many years, researchers have speculated on whether humans have the ability to detect pheromones; the phenomenon that the menstrual cycles of women who live together change gradually and involuntarily until they are in sync seems to provide evidence that pheromones exist and that they can indeed influence people. The so-called *McClintock effect* proves that underarm swabs collected from female donors, when whipped under the noses of other women, influence cycle length and timing and, furthermore, that exposure to male axillary (armpit) extracts can normalize irregular menstrual cycles.

The smell of a baby's cuddly body or freshly baked bread, the musty scent of an eighteenth-century book, or the earthy aroma of a rainy day are equal in their uniqueness—and vaginas are no exception. As with any great perfume counter, there is a vast array of scents emitting from our lovely lady parts: Whether it is nondescript, a fruity or floral scent, a warm earthy bouquet, or a seductively spicy, oriental aroma, it is unique and unforgettable. There is absolutely nothing to be anxious about as far as our vaginal odor goes; it is our own intimate or shared secret, an enchanting whisper rather than a blatant announcement. Dearest fellow Eves, whether we smell like jasmine, cinnamon, or alfalfa sprouts, be assured that vaginal odor is hardly unappealing—quite the contrary.

MANIPULATING THE SMELL OF YOUR POSY

Although feminine odor is quite unique to every individual, there are a number of lifestyle factors that can directly influence our intimate aroma. When we opt for the healthier route we will be amazed at the lovely effect that it has on our hidden treasure.

Scents and Sensibility

We are well aware of the importance of hygiene: If we don't wash ourselves regularly, we will certainly not come up smelling like roses. The apocrine sweat glands found in hair follicles in the armpits, around the nipples, and in our pubic region release secretions that consist of an unscented solution made up of 99 percent water. Emotional stress, sexual excitement, heat, and exercise trigger these secretions, and if your body is left unwashed after an active day, you are bound to smell quite questionable. A simple, daily wash with a color- and fragrance-free soap, or a natural product like a tea tree intimate wash, will help destroy pesky odor-producing bacteria on the vulva and prevent any unpleasant scents from developing in that region.

Your showerhead is a tool you can use to introduce water to all your external nooks and crannies, or you can run a bath and use your fingers to gently cleanse your labia. There is no need whatsoever to spray anything on your intimate bits. Not only is it unnecessary, but it can also be extremely harmful as the vaginal crevice is completely self-cleansing. Douching, which entails applying a jet of water inside the vagina, is generally a big no-no since it can, much to our dismay, increase discharge and bad odor by upsetting the sensitive vaginal ecosystem and may even cause pelvic inflammation. Douching should be done only when prescribed by a medical doctor.

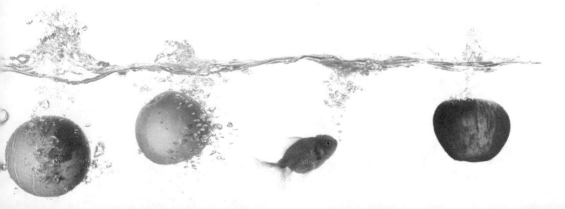

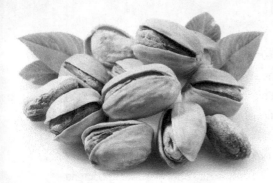

On that note, here is a charming but ludicrous excerpt from a book written by a Dr. H. H. Rubin in 1938: "One very frequent reason for men making extra-marital alliances is because of the fact that the odor that emanates from the body of the wife—particularly if the husband and wife should foolishly share the same bed—is so obnoxious that it destroys all appetite for closer contact. If a woman has a tendency toward any vaginal discharge she should use a vaginal douche morning and night until this condition is thoroughly cleared up." At least now we know better, and hopefully we are "foolish" enough to share and enjoy the same bed with our beloved!

It is also important to remember to change tampons and diaphragms regularly: If left in for too long, either product can cause our nether regions to emit a most unattractive odor. It makes "scents"; doesn't it?

Cookies and Cuisine

Indulging in garlic, onions, and hot spices will cause many smells to ooze from our pores, and this applies to our intimate fragrance as well. Drinking alcohol like a fish could also cause our vaginas to smell, well, much like a fish.

When we do need a sweet release, which usually comes in the form of some kind of chocolaty substance, moderation is the key. Cigarettes, too many fizzy drinks, or an excess of red meat and coffee also affect the odor department and are definite no-nos. We may wilt in the face of our temptations, but beware. These harmful delights will make the scent from our vaginas more acidic and sharp to the nose.

Be brave and inquisitive enough to poke your nose into your own business: Monitor your aroma to see what affect the food and drink you are consuming has on your vaginal odor. Seafood such as crayfish is known to cause a sweet smell, and a diet that includes tropical fruit such as papaya can create a soft, fruity aroma. Eat as naturally and as healthfully as possible, drink plenty of water, and have a spoonful of alkaline powder daily (available at health-food stores and pharmacies) to balance your body's pH. The change will be delightfully apparent. As they say, the proof is in the pudding!

Changes During Our Cycle

Ladies whose bodies have not yet made their menopausal announcements, and those who are not on the Pill, will experience variations in the odor department during their cycle—as the pH or acidity balance of the vagina changes, so does the smell. Both men and women can distinguish between the olfactory clues that the body emits during the phases of our cycle. During ovulation (the reproductive phase), the scent of Eros spices up our vaginal odors to lure prospective suitors to our honey pot. In Pill users, the attractiveness ratings of our intimate odors do not differ significantly during the cycle, which is not to say that an oral contraceptive makes odors less attractive but merely that it cancels the rhythmic fragrance changes of our lady parts.

Kohl and Francoeur offer good news on our ability to detect smells. They state, under the fabulous heading, "The Natural Superiority of Women," that since men have high levels of testosterone, which inhibits and diminishes the sense of smell, they have a much poorer perception of odors than women. Women, who have increased levels of estrogen, are naturally equipped with

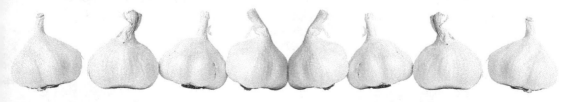

an acute sense of smell. After puberty, we are a one hundred times more sensitive to certain smells than our male counterparts. Furthermore, when we ovulate, our sensitivity increases by up to a hundred thousand-fold! Although we are, for instance, aware of the earthy aroma of menstrual fluid during the menstrual phase of our cycle, there is absolutely no need to be oversensitive to our vaginal aromas. Period.

Between the Sheets

Thoughts of an intelligible nature are generally few and far between during our moments of bedroom bliss; thinking about avoiding contamination of the vagina with organisms from the rectum is hardly at the top of one's list. Be that as it may, it is extremely important to prevent such contamination.

If you don't know your partner very well, never, ever consider engaging in unprotected sex; condoms are essential in preventing sexually transmitted infections, which are, in most cases, faithfully accompanied by unpleasant smells. To ensure that you remain safe and sound and alive, please don't treat this in a lighthearted, devil-may-care manner; an unwrapped candle is most definitely not worth the cake.

When it comes to vaginal odor, unprotected sex also means a change in your intimate aroma. A healthy vagina has a pH of 3.8 to 4.5, which means that it is slightly acidic. This creates a perfect environment that serves as a natural defense enhancer to ward off infections. Semen, on the other hand, has a very high alkaline level (a pH count of 7.4 to 8.0) and after unprotected intercourse, the pH level of the vagina escalates for up to twenty-four hours, which not only makes it more vulnerable to infections but also increases the potency of its smell. This can make the morning-after thrill not so thrilling after all!

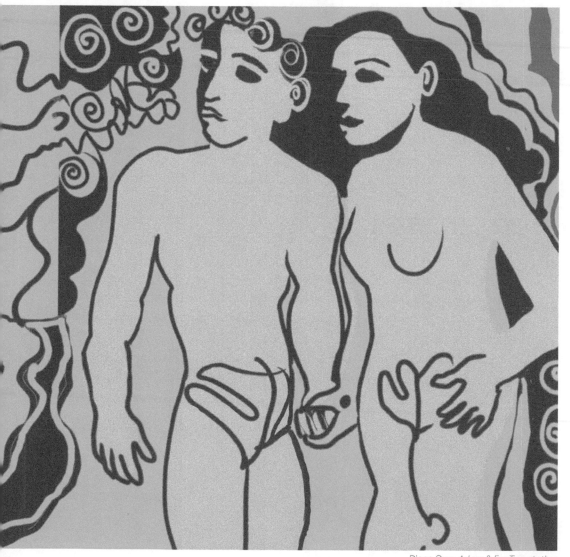

Diana Ong, *Adam & Eve Temptation*

CHAPTER 4

SNATCH 22: HONEY POT OR HINDRANCE?

The thought of a vagina certainly evokes a number of images and ideas in the minds of both men and women. Often this thought is tainted by feelings of anxiety and viewed as a subject to be found in the heart of society's taboos. Men feel intimidated, both awed and strangely appalled by the sheer power of it.

Shrouded in mystery, the vagina, among its many glorious achievements, has the power to give birth to another human being, and any man who has experienced such an event certainly doesn't leave the birthing room the same man as when he entered. We, on the other hand, often wonder if having the father of our children witness our giving birth might blemish our future sex life.

Furthermore, at some time or another we feel ashamed and abashed, concerned with the look, the smell, and perhaps the taste of our vaginas. And then, of course, once a month we are reacquainted with our menstrual period, which can be an occurrence equally alarming for both men and women — not to mention an inconvenience when we go on a hiking or camping trip. From a social and practical point of view, we also, contrary to our male counterparts, miss out on the convenience of urinating while standing or having a collective wee-wee outside with our girlfriends on a moonlit evening. Then there's the dreaded, distressing visit to the gynecologist, which women must suffer annually. We strip down, feeling anxious and self-conscious about a plethora of things; from the cleanliness of our lady parts to the inevitability of pain, to the possibility that there might be something wrong with our vaginas and, therefore, our health. There is also a link between feeling physically awkward and feeling emotionally defenseless. After all, our pretty intimates are not often exposed, and thus we experience feelings of immense vulnerability.

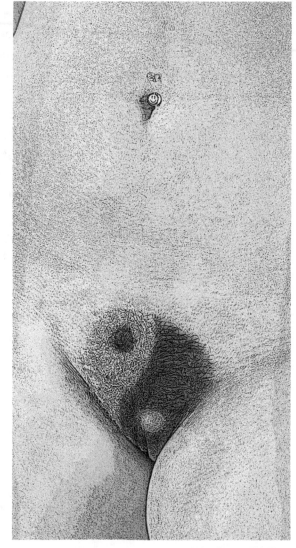

Milan Cronje, *Ying Yang*

But then again, the vagina is a gift of beauty and strength, a vault of endless pleasures, a treasure trove. It has the power to bring grown men to their knees—quite literally! Women who wholeheartedly embrace their femininity and sexuality proudly describe their vaginas as "extraordinarily beautiful," "magnificent," and "marvelous."

It is quite normal to hold both negative and positive views concerning our lady parts, and although having a vagina does not necessarily, apart from our anatomy, define us as women, this trait does unite us in our womanhood, and that is something to celebrate. Knowledge and awareness concerning the changes that our vaginas go through regarding their appearances, odors, tastes, and secretions are paramount for self-awareness and can free us from the unnecessary anxieties we harbor.

Change is in our hands: When we view our vaginas as sources of pride and wonder rather than something of which to be ashamed, we empower ourselves beyond question. If we declare our suppressed and silent views by recognizing ourselves as the agents and speakers for and creators of our intimate worlds, then this secret, sensuous place—the one brimming with pleasures—is a benefit if ever there was one. When we take pride in our bodies and project strong sexual identities, we can most certainly derive much fulfillment and joy from our private and shared experiences.

In order for the human race to continue, women must be safe and empowered.
It's an obvious idea, but like a vagina, it needs great attention and love in order to be revealed.

— Eve Ensler

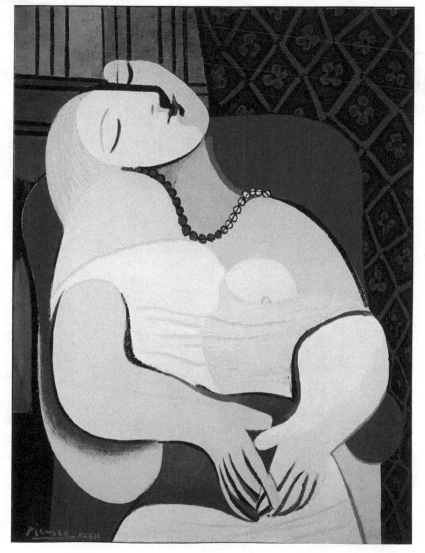

Pablo Picasso, *The Dream*

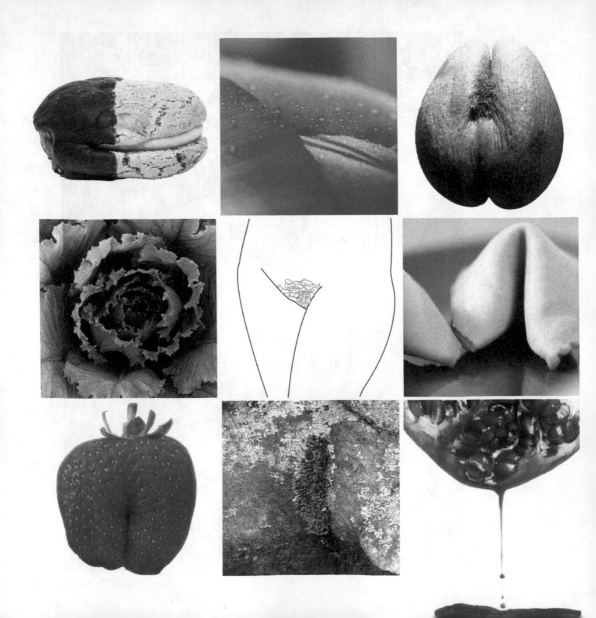

PART II

FLOWER POWER:
LIVING WITH A VAGINA

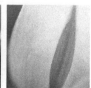

CHAPTER 5

KITTY CORNER

What are little girls made of?
What are little girls made of?
Sugar and spice and all things nice,
That's what little girls are made of.

When we look at the differences between boys and girls, we find that much of boys' sexual identification is linked to the fact that they have a penis. Parents often express appreciation and praise when their two-year-old son flaunts his penis; this gives the proud boy the notion that he is the owner of a priceless body part. The penis is truly a wonderful object; a natural little plaything, it is able to launch an entertaining stream of urine that can be proudly sprayed and splashed around while standing. This tool can also be used as a weapon, and a little boy might provoke siblings by literally "pissing them off."

For little girls, however, a vagina is her secret organ. Not only is it invisible to her, but it is also often viewed in a negative light if touched by her, and "whatchamacallit" code words and

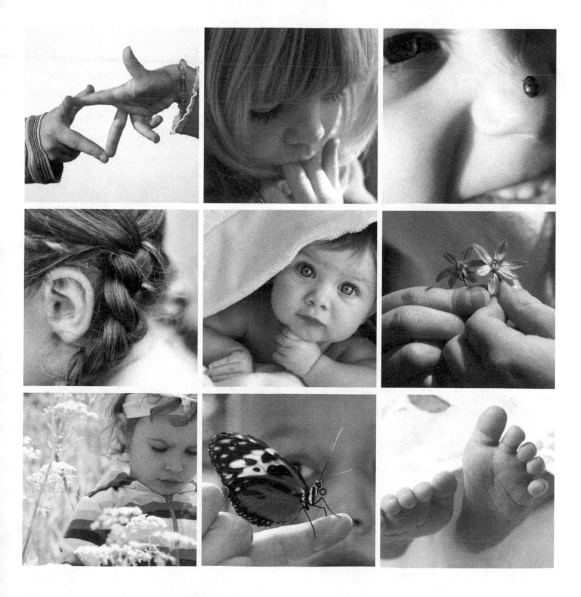

euphemisms further aid in neatly concealing this hidden treasure. When nature calls for desperate measures, she has to hide and crouch to urinate—an inconvenient and often embarrassing affair. Boys understand from an early stage that privacy and shame are two separate concepts: They learn to be both proud and private with regard to their genitalia. For young girls, the mysteriousness and privacy of their genitalia are often veiled in secrecy and shame. This disparity in underlying values is carried with us well into adulthood and can have a significant influence on our sexual health. From this point of view, it appears that women start off with a disadvantage that gives us even more reason to invite some change.

GENITAL FONDLING

The famous human sexual response researcher William Masters (1925–2001), an American gynecologist, was known to play a game with newborn boys during delivery, saying "Can I get the cord cut before the kid has an erection?" But he often failed since most boys are born with a fully erect penis. He also observed that all baby girls lubricated vaginally in the first four to six hours of life, and that during sleep, spontaneous erections or vaginal lubrication occur every eighty to ninety minutes throughout our entire life span.

Despite being born with sexuality as an inherent part of a child's being, expressions of a sexual nature often leave parents with a feeling of discomfort and concern. "Sexual nature" in this context refers to behavior that includes touching, sexual identification, exploring one's own body and those of others, sexual language, masturbation, and games or interaction that have sexual connotations. Although children vary in their interest in sexuality, they are all naturally curious about their own bodies and those of others. Investigative peeking games that entail *"you-show-me-yours-and-I'll-show-you-mine"* are quite natural.

Yes, moms and dads, if you are one of the 85 percent of people who "played doctor" when you were between the ages of three and seven, you will, in all probability, know exactly what we are talking about. For those who have missed out on this adventurous, albeit "naughty" game, "playing doctor" is a colloquial phrase that refers to the incidence of children engaging in the examination of one another's genitals. Rest assured that these games are considered normal and are viewed as nonsexual behavior.

Caught with Your Hand in the Cookie Jar?

It is also well known that, girls discover their magic buttons of pleasure whether or not they play *peek-a-boo* with others. A girl may become aware of a pleasurable sensation caused by the friction of her underwear, riding on her bicycle, climbing ropes or trees, or gently rocking or rubbing her teddy bear between her legs.

Masturbation is such a weighty word to use when talking about our innocent girl children, and although polite society doesn't freely discuss matters of such delicacy, we should realize that it is quite a natural, nonsexual occurrence. Her private enjoyment of self-stimulation should be viewed in the light and innocent character of all childish diversions. You may find that she masturbates when she is tired, bored, or simply relaxing. Perhaps all we need to do is explain to our little girl that it is a private matter, and as long as she doesn't pick the supermarket, the neighbors' Sunday barbeque, or the beachfront for private playtime, all is well.

To illustrate this principle, we have a lovely account of a father reading a bedtime story to his twenty-month-old little girl. Sophie would sometimes enjoy her "happy wiggle" as she relaxed and listened to the calm and comforting voice of her father. In these instances, her dad would pause and say, "Do you want to be alone, or do you want to hear the story?" Although worried about Sophie's behavior at first, her parents found that once they had discussed this openly and

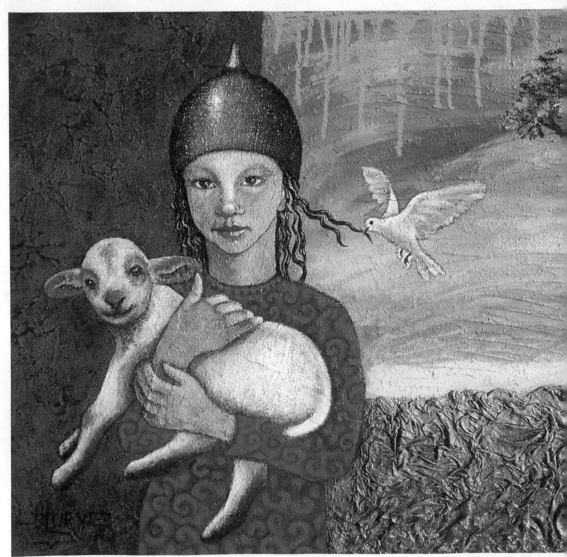

Helen Lurye, *Army of One*

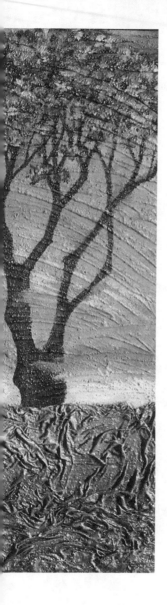

told her it was something she should do in private, it stopped being such a big deal. Notably, Sophie was educated in a positive way without leaving her with feelings of guilt and shame.

Well worth mentioning, too, is certain sexual behavior girls may exhibit that merits some reason for concern. This includes attempting or imitating sexual intercourse with a friend, dolls, or other soft toys; attempts to insert objects into her own or a friend's anus or vagina; oral–genital contact; demanding that others take part in explicit sexual activities; and obsessive self-stimulation. Based on the fact that these tendencies are uncommon in emotionally healthy children but common among children who have been victims of abuse, these deviances require adult intervention.

Please listen when little ones talk about things that seem grown-up and removed from their frame of reference. They do not have the cognitive capabilities to talk about sexual acts unless they've experienced them. Symptoms of possible abuse include a change in behavior that reveals anger, hostility, aggression, or withdrawal; nightmares; bed-wetting and fear of the dark; regression to babyish habits; or displaying reticence toward or fear of a person or a situation. School grades and attention span may also be affected.

Since we are on the topic of masturbation, let us linger a little longer before we return to our little girls and their vaginas. A clay figurine from a temple site on the island of Malta, dating back to the fourth millennium BC, depicts a woman masturbating, providing evidence that this private delight has been around for many a year. During the Victorian Era, however, there was such widespread medical and social censure of masturbation that boys' trousers were designed in such a way that the genitals could not be touched through the pockets and girls were forbidden to sit cross-legged or ride horses and bicycles. Children who continued to indulge in these practices were branded as "weak-minded," and remedies like eating a bland, meatless diet were devised to stop this behavior.

Dr. John Harvey Kellogg (1852–1943), an American medical doctor and the brother of the brainchild of *"You got it all this morning"* Corn Flakes, was a huge supporter of this "bland diet" idea. He suggested that the "terribly evil vice" of genital fondling be cured by fully occupying a child with work or activities so that he will be too tired to have the inclination to "defile" himself. He further advised placing a child under twenty-four-hour surveillance; bandaging the genital parts; tying the hands and covering the organs with a cage at night; preventing erections by putting a silver wire through the skin on either side of the penis and twisting the ends together in such a way as to draw the two sides closely together, and performing circumcision without anesthetic to have an everlasting salutary effect upon the boy's mind. For little girls, Dr. Kellogg recommended the application of pure carbolic acid to the clitoris as an "excellent" means of allaying the "abnormal excitement."

Other Victorian preventative procedures to discourage masturbation included electroshock treatment, wearing chastity belts and straitjackets, and, ultimately, extensive surgical excision of the genitals! In later years, psychological techniques were used to warn against masturbation. If you are my age, you may remember the warning that masturbation would result in "blindness, hairy hands, and stunted growth."

According to Dr. Kellogg, the warning signs of childhood masturbation included seeing "the roses leave their cheeks, the luster depart from their eyes, the elasticity from their step, the glow of health and purity from their faces, increasing languor and lassitude, causing the poor victim to drop into a premature grave."

Apart from death, symptoms further included back aches, spinal diseases, memory loss, ulcers on the fingertips, pimples, hysteria, bed-wetting, loss of appetite, swelling of the legs, epilepsy, gout, rheumatism, and blood in the urine. Consequently, the person "becomes a mere animal, who eats, sleeps, and breathes; utterly deprived of all human characteristics. He is conscious of neither joy nor grief, pleasure nor pain. He sits staring vacantly into space, with an open, drooling mouth, and a senseless, idiotic smile upon his face."

Fortunately, these negative views began to change at the beginning of the twentieth century when H. Havelock Ellis, pioneer British sexologist (1859–1939), saved us from a life of "blandness." He firmly points out that the misguided notions of many unscrupulous quacks caused the suffering, dread, and remorse experienced in silence

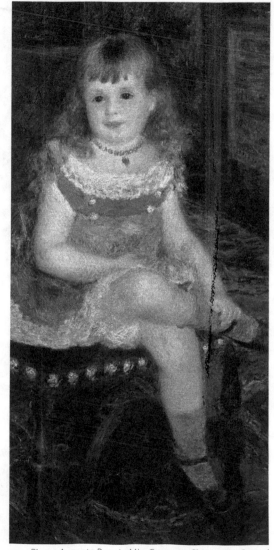

Pierre-Auguste Renoir, *Miss Georgette Charpentier Seated*

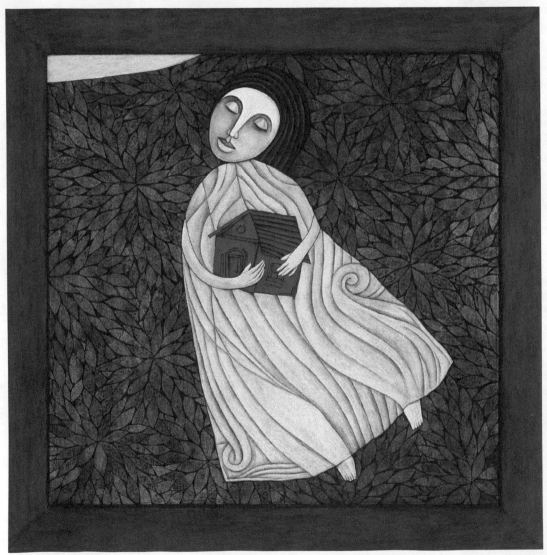

Daniel Nevins, *So Close*

by many thousands of ignorant and often innocent young people, and states that "with moderate masturbation in healthy, well-born Individuals, no seriously pernicious results necessarily follow."

Today we know that masturbation holds a wide range of health benefits. It helps prevent and relieve cervical inflammation and urinary tract infections; improves cardiovascular health and lowers the risk of type-2 diabetes; relieves insomnia, stress, and anxiety; strengthens the muscles of our pelvic floor; is a natural mood booster; helps people who do not have an available partner to maintain sexual functioning and expression; aids in sexual intimacy and satisfaction within relationships; and enhances feelings of self love and body awareness that contribute to a sense of ownership, control, and autonomy. We can safely say that joy in a natural, beneficial, and healthy way is only a "happy wiggle" away, but of course not all itches are pleasant....

"MOMMY, I HAVE AN ITCH!"

Reassuringly, it is not unusual for our little ones to experience irritation and discomfort in the vaginal region. The most common complaints include:
- a painful vagina with no redness or itchiness
- a sore, itchy vagina that looks slightly red with no discharge
- a sore, itchy vagina with a whitish discharge or white spots (tiny blisters) sitting in the folds and/or around the outside of the vagina
- discomfort when urinating

And the most likely causes include:
- sweat and friction

- vaginal infections such as a yeast infection (thrush) or bacterial vaginosis

- an allergic reaction

- a foreign object in the vagina

- sexual abuse

Tight-fitting clothes and synthetic underwear create friction and sweating, which may cause vaginal soreness and induce secondary bacterial infection. Diapers, which can be a source of both heat and moisture, also create an environment that encourages fungal growth, so it is best to change diapers frequently.

Vaginitis (inflammation of the vagina) is usually caused by infections like thrush and bacterial vaginosis. To identify thrush (a yeast infection), watch for a white, cottage cheese–like discharge, itching, and irritated skin; this can be remedied with an over-the-counter, antifungal clotrimazole cream. Bacterial vaginosis causes itching and burning, and the key identifier here is a fishy odor. In this case, it is sensible to be lead by the nose: You'll need to take your little girl to the doctor, since she needs to be treated with antibiotics. Allergic reactions can be caused by perfumed soaps, bubble baths, colored and perfumed toilet paper, and nylon undies — all of which are certainly worth avoiding if you discover they tend to be a problem.

Lastly, little girls have been known to insert anything from pieces of toilet paper to small toys, cheese curls, or peas into their vaginas, and such foreign objects can cause a very smelly and offensive discharge. If you discover your daughter has inserted something into her vagina, you can try to remove it yourself before calling the doctor. Have her stand with one leg elevated, let's say, on the toilet-seat. With clean hands, gently try to remove the foreign matter. If this exercise is too traumatic for mother or child, it is best to consult a doctor.

Moms and dads, here is our plan of action to help our little ones maintain a healthy vagina. If we follow these basic guidelines, we'll keep our kittens untroubled and happily purring away:

- Change your baby's diapers regularly.
- Avoid scented or colored toilet paper and creams. Save the bubble bath for special occasions.
- Use warm water and an unscented "soft" soap, such as Elizabeth Anne's, to clean the genital area once a day
- Teach your little girl to always wipe from front to back.
- Have her wear cotton underwear and change her underwear daily.
- Encourage her to wear loose-fitting clothing to allow this sensitive area to remain as cool and chafe-free as possible.
- Do not let her play in a swimsuit all day long.
- If she experiences recurring thrush, make an appointment with the doctor. Have the doctor take a swab from her vagina to determine the exact cause of the infection.
- Be aware of urinary tract infections (UTIs), as they are quite common in little girls. If you suspect a UTI (burning or pain with urination), consult your doctor.

CHAPTER 6

FROM TOT TO TEEN

PUBERTY

Puberty follows a reasonably consistent sequence in girls. At a quick glance, this is what you can expect:

- Breast buds develop. This can occur any time between the ages of seven and thirteen.

- Coarse, dark hair appears under the arms and on the labia majora. About 15 percent of girls develop the pubic hair first and then the bee stings.

- The first menstrual cycle occurs, on average, around 2 to 2½ years after the onset of breast development. Although 12.6 years is the average age for a first menstrual period, anything from age 9 to 15 is considered standard. Generally women get their period every 28 days, but an interval of 21 days up to 40 days is also viewed as normal.

As girls begin to produce increasing levels of estrogen, the mucosal surface of their girly-parts starts to change color. The prepubertal mucosa has a bright red tinge and will, with the onset of puberty, become thicker and turn a paler pink. Another telltale sign that your girl is

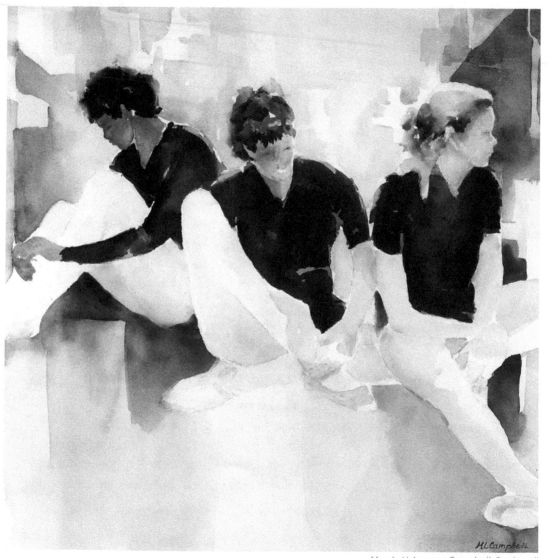

Margie Livingston Campbell, *Entr'acte II*

about to have her first period is a whitish, odorless vaginal discharge. This secretion is called *leucorrhea* and is a normal indicator that hormonal changes are taking place. Leucorrhea is part of the vagina's natural defense mechanism to maintain a healthy chemical balance, and it also preserves vaginal tissue flexibility. As a matter of general interest, let us look at factors that influence a girls' first menstrual period, also known as *menarche* (**me**-náar-ki).

First and foremost, the mother's history and her age at onset of menstruation offer the strongest predictor of a girl's first period. The next biggest factor is harmony within the family circle: Girls who are exposed to high-conflict family relationships (including poverty and parental neglect) tend to mature earlier. Girls who grow up in warm, supportive, low-stress environments with close and meaningful relationships with family members also enjoy longer grace periods to remain girly and carefree as menarche is delayed. In extremely stressful situations such as wartime, undernourishment, or sexual abuse, however, the body experiences a threat to physical survival, causing the puberty process to be delayed.

A very interesting and strong determining factor of menarche timing lies in the father–daughter relationship. Girls are very sensitive to the quality of paternal care they receive, and it directly affects their sexual development. Fatherly affection and involvement, for instance, relate to later onset, and although the death of a loving father has no influence on menarche, the absence of a biological father through separation or divorce is known to accelerate the arrival of the first menstrual period.

Fathers who carry the shorter alleles of the androgen receptor (AR) gene are more likely to abandon a marriage, and this gene is genetically passed on to their daughters in whom it produces an earlier age of menarche. Sadly, divorce or separation in a child's formative years predicts not only early menarche but also early sexual intercourse, early pregnancy, and high counts of sexual partners.

Another equally strong predicative factor is the presence of a stepfather. This correlates to the "male effect," a phenomenon found in a variety of mammals that demonstrates accelerated onset of menarche when unrelated adult males are introduced into a colony. The last significant factor that triggers early menarche is obesity: When a young girl's body mass reaches $\pm$ 110 pounds, it may initiate the menstruation process.

MENSTRUATION

The first day of red or brownish spotting is to be remembered for a very long time. This is an exciting time, but sadly it is often clouded by fear, secrecy, and embarrassment. Open and positive communication between mothers and daughters is of paramount importance during this time, as the messages received from Mom will play the biggest role in our daughters' first-time experience and overall view of becoming a woman. Expressions such as "the curse," "on the rag," "the weeping womb," "bloody scourge," and "the red plague" are bound to instill fear, disgust, and negativity. Archaic notions that menstruation is dangerous; that it contaminates crops, tribes, food and wine; that it brings bad luck to the hunter; or that "bleeding" women should be excluded from worship, must clearly be ignored.

In too many cases, mothers fail to talk to their daughters and neglect to offer emotional support with regard to changing relationships with parents, siblings, and friends. Secrecy around carrying, storing, using, and discarding menstrual products is also often implied. Only 15 percent of young ladies report a positive first-time experience; 68 percent have no awareness of their mother's experience with menstruation and 64 percent receive negative messages from their mothers. As girls move toward this rite of passage, it provides us with an ideal platform to strengthen the special mother–daughter bond.

During menstruation our young ladies may become irritable or suffer headaches, tiredness, and premenstrual pain. Premenstrual pain has been part of being a woman since the dawn of time. It can be an agonizingly uncomfortable experience, and those who have suffered the discomfort and pain are not likely to forget it, while those who no longer suffer from it are as unlikely to mourn its absence.

Some women and girls have compared this pain to hot coals in the stomach; some experience a dull ache in the lower back and weakness of the legs; others equate it to a slightly milder version of labor pains. Please assure your daughter that it is all a normal part of growing up and give her something for the pain. Some prescription-only medication can be taken, but over-the-counter tablets like ibuprofen and naproxen also can be extremely effective in washing the pain away.

To say that losing a few tablespoons of blood once a month (in actual fact, approximately ¼ cup/2 ounces) is "uncomfortable and inconvenient" is an understatement. We all know what an ambitious task it can be to keep a bright mood during this time. Despite all the facts to the contrary, menstruation pain (or *dysmenorrhoea*) isn't all bad; believe it or not, there are perks, albeit very few, but perks nonetheless. We can take some pleasure in the pain by indulging in many a guilty delight—I find the sweeter the delectation the better. Menstruation can also give us an excuse to stay in bed and distract ourselves with ice cream and a good, old-fashioned, romantic movie. Whether we are writhing in agony or simply lying on our beds, clutching a hot water bottle for dear life, we can take comfort in the fact that we are certainly not alone in our misery. The fact that this pain is unique to the fairer sex and experienced by every woman at one time or another is something quite special. Apart from allowing us some "down time," this experience binds us together in a shared sisterhood.

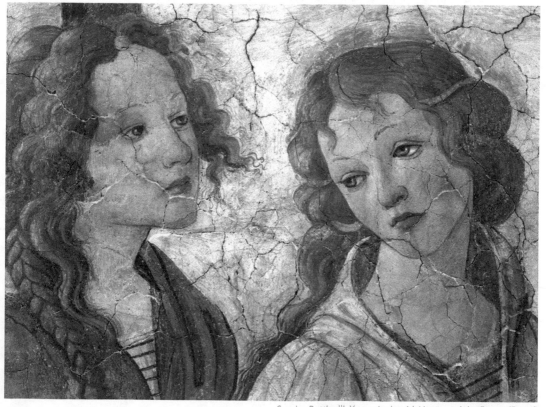

Sandro Botticelli, *Young Lady with Venus and the Graces (Detail)*

Celebrating Menarche

Menarche celebrations around the world confirm the importance of this huge step into womanhood. In Australia, an Aborigine girl is instructed in "love magic" and taught the female powers of being a woman. Love magic rituals are designed to attract a targeted marriage partner or someone suitable for a sexual liaison. Singing and dancing over a strand of hair of the desired mate or dropping a string tied with feathers into the prospective partner's basket is said to ignite the most irresistible desire.

In Japan, the entire family celebrates a girl's first period by eating red-colored rice and beans. In Sri Lanka, this special time and day are noted, and an astrologer is contacted to study the stars' alignment and predict the girl's future. Her house is prepared for a ritual bathing, and the girl is scrubbed from head to toe by the women of the family and then dressed in white. Printed invitations are sent out for a party, during which the girl receives money and special gifts.

In rural India, a girl who has reached puberty is given a ceremonial bath and adorned with ornate jewels and garments, and the girl's friends and family are invited for a festive ceremony. In Kumari, Nepal, the young girls are worshipped as goddesses, and Nootka Indians believe menarche to be a time to test a girl's physical strength and endurance: She is taken out to sea and left alone in the water. The girl has to swim back and is cheered upon returning to the shore of the village.

The Mescalero Apaches consider their menarche celebration the most important event on the calendar. Each year, an eight-day-long ceremony is held in honor of every girl who has started her period during that year. The first four days are spent feasting and dancing, and each evening boy singers recount the history of the tribe. The following four days are devoted to a celebration during which girls have a private ceremony and reflect on their entrance into womanhood. The following song of rejoicing signals the end of the maturation celebration of these girls:

Now you are entering the world.
You will become an adult with responsibilities…
Walk with honor and dignity.
Be strong!
For you are the mother of our people…
For you will become the mother of a nation.

Wonderful! Don't you think that it is a brilliant idea to do something really special too for your girl(s) as they join us and share the solidarity among women? Be it a private diary to record her experiences as a woman, a special calendar to mark the frequency of her menstrual cycle, pierced ears or a first leg-shave, a new nightgown, or a shared outing, let the prospect of her first period be something wondrous and exciting for her to anticipate. Talk to her and explain what is about to happen, and let her be equipped by preparing a special toiletry bag for school: Pack an extra pair of underwear and a pad or two, and surprise her with a small "welcome-to-womanhood" gift. Good luck!

CHAPTER 7

ON VIRGIN TERRITORY

"Unashamedly" retrieved from poet Polly Kitzinger's wastepaper basket by her mother, Sheila Kitzinger, the author of *Woman's Experience of Sex* (1983), the following poem illustrates the developmental phase during which young women start to break away from being clones of their moms in an attempt to claim the boundaries of their own identity:

Mother, Mother, Mother-goddess,
moulding your child into beauty,
You take her by the hand
And lead her gently into life,
Your beautiful daughter
Into your beautiful life.
There is nothing she can do
That you cannot accept, understand, forgive,
There is nothing she can do.

There is nothing she can be
That you will not re-interpret into beauty
There is nothing I can be,
Mother, Mother, Mother,
I am screaming
Let me be.
Do not come into my room, Mother,
Do not come and make it beautiful and fresh
with your flowers and your love,
Do not breathe into it your love of life,
Your joy, your joyful view of life,
Here in my dark stale room I sit alone
amongst the crumbs, the coffee-cups, the smelly socks
I pick my nose, I lick my plate,
Hugging my sordid individuality about me
Like barbed wire
Keeping you out
I am I, not she—your daughter,
I am Me.

— Polly Kitzinger

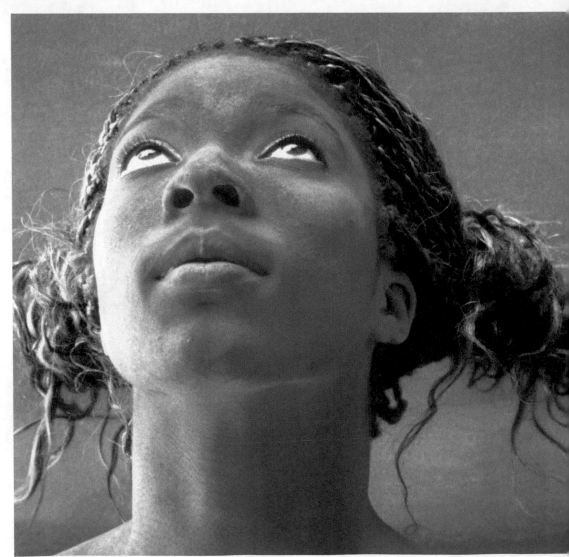

Filippo ioco, *Midnight Swim*

It is quite natural for young women to entertain the thought of sexual intercourse. The concept of "virginity," a treasured aspect of our being, now comes to the fore, and since it is closely associated with the perforation of the hymen (or the maidenhead), this thin fold of mucous membrane merits closer examination.

THE MYSTICAL MAIDENHEAD

> *De hymenis existentia nemo dubitat.*
> *[No one doubts the existence of the hymen.]*
> — Brendelius, eighteenth-century forensic anatomist

We are all born with a hymen, but the variations in shape and thickness can be considerable. It can leave the entrance to the vagina completely unobstructed or block it entirely (a medical condition called the *imperforate hymen*). Although there is no known physical function of the hymen, research shows that it is an embryological structure with the sole purpose to protect the vagina against infection during infancy. It then remains in place well into the adolescent years. Once a girl reaches puberty, the hymen tends to be so elastic that only 43 percent of women report bleeding the first time they have sexual intercourse.

This indicates that the vaginal crevice is sufficiently opened and supple enough to allow for penile penetration. Subsequently, even if the hymen is intact, no one can predict if defloration (tearing of the hymen) will be accompanied with blood loss. Testosterone-fuelled juveniles, preoccupied with sexual conquests and dreaming about "*popping a girl's cherry*" (to use more vernacular language), will in all probability be disappointed.

Many women tear or stretch their hymens through physical activities such as bike riding, gymnastics, or other athletics, while the hymens of others remain intact notwithstanding sexual experimentation. Interestingly, 52 percent of women who have experienced penile penetration still have a "nondisrupted" hymen, and up to 64 percent of adolescents' hymens remain intact during pregnancy. Although the presence, absence, or the physical appearance of the hymen reveals very little about a woman's sexual experience, its psychological and cultural significance as a sign of virginity is still of critical importance in many societies.

A virgin (or maiden) refers to a woman who has never had sexual intercourse. The word derives from the Latin *virgo*, which means "sexually inexperienced woman." We place a high premium on our virginity, and unlike men, who can literally wash-up and wash-off after having had sexual intercourse (not to claim that intercourse has little or no effect on men), we are unable, on both a physical and emotional level, to "wash out" this intimate invasion we so passionately allow. This necessitates that we carefully calibrate this degree of intimacy to ensure that it leaves us with cherished memories.

In some cultural groups, however, the loss of virginity extends beyond the personal sphere and manifests itself deeply in the heart of a much broader power dynamic. "Shame-based" patriarchal societies implement "proof of virginity" measures to control women's sexuality and to repress their role in society. Women who have lost their virginity before marriage are vulnerable to emotional and physical torture, jail sentencing, or even death under the rubric of "crimes of honor."

The presentation of a virginity certificate or the presence of a bloodstained sheet serves as proof of a bride's virginity, while it assures the bridegroom's parents that the young woman is well worth the "bride price." In Tunisia, for instance, the bride-to-be will make an appointment with a medical doctor for an *el certifikka sbiyya* (a virginity certificate) before the signing of the marriage contract.

On the long-awaited wedding night, while the bridegroom delights in deflowering his bride, apprehensive guests wait eagerly to see the bloodstained sheet. She saves her sheet carefully for the show-and-tell session, and if the stain remains bright pink, pale pink, or scarlet, she will be swollen with pride for years to come. The bloodstained sheet is also believed to contain magical powers: Not only is it a sign that the young woman is endowed with wisdom, but it is also alleged that the mere sight of the bloodied sheet will protect the elderly from blindness.

In rural Egypt, the deliberate tearing of the hymen is performed during a defloration ritual on the wedding day. A *daya,* the same woman who performs the circumcision of the girls, keeps one of her fingernails long and sharp for this occasion. If she lacerates the hymen and the wall of the vagina, which causes more blood to flow onto the white sheet (to be paraded by the father of the bride), her work is considered most successful. OUCH! Just imagine the dangerous infections this ritual can cause.

In Southern Africa, "virginity testing" is a longstanding custom among the Zulu and, to a lesser extent, the Xhosa tribes. This controversial and potentially dangerous practice is addressed in The South African Children's Act No. 38 of 2005 — traditional circumcision and virginity testing are permitted after the age of sixteen, but only with the girl's consent and after she has received counseling. The bill also prescribes that the results of the test may not be disclosed without the permission of the child, nor may she be identified in any way. Unfortunately, these prescriptions go unheeded, and the practice seems to be gaining momentum. Girls as young as six years of age are exposed to unhygienic and degrading physical inspections, which are often carried out in front of large crowds. Some girls place toothpaste, lace, or freshly cut meat in their vaginal canal for it to appear tighter and to resemble an untouched, virginal vagina.

Equally contentious is the claim that boys, too, have hymens. As we witness the birth of yet another false belief, this assertion continues to gain support in attempts to certify boy virgins. It is maintained that a boy's hymen is white and lacy, and if the foreskin slips easily and painlessly over the tip of the penis, the hymen is broken and the boy a virgin no longer. Other telltale signs of a male's "broken hymen" include not being able to urinate straight up into the air, an inability to urinate without spraying, and the evidence of a darker skin color around the knees.

Faking It: Having a Second "First Time"

Since the proof of a young woman's maidenhood determines a woman's value and status in some societies, many resort to deception or a procedure called "hymenoplasty" to disguise a broken hymen. Often deception involves the use of chicken blood or a small cut to the finger to produce a stain on the wedding sheet to create the illusion of virginity.

Hymen repair also has a long history: Midwives disguised a broken hymen by attaching membranes from goats and other animals, with a needle and thread, to the opening of the vagina. Today, however, you can have a thirty-minute outpatient procedure — one semicircular cut, ten dissolving stitches later — and *voilà,* your odometer is turned back to zero! During these procedures, the vaginal wall is stitched together from the left to the right to ensure that upon entry of the penis, tearing of the mucous membrane is guaranteed.

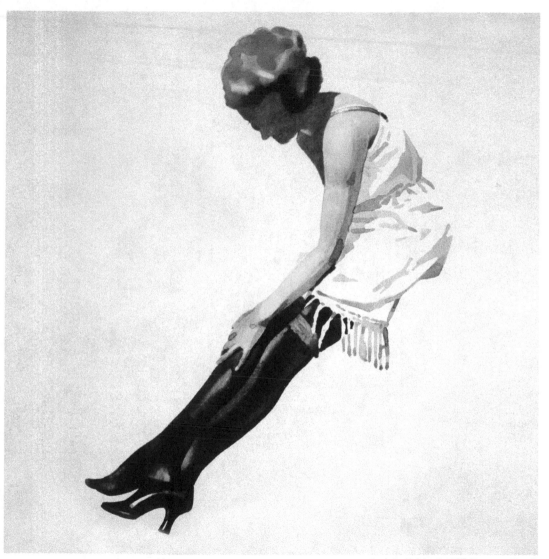

Ludwig Hohlwein, *LBO Damenstrümpfe*

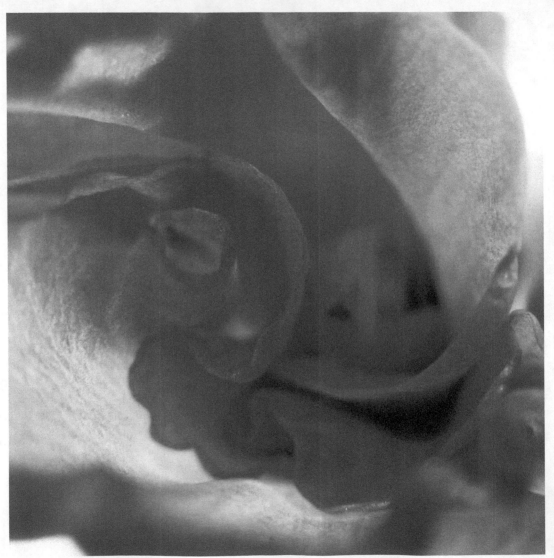

Teresa Jeffcote, *Delicate*

Whether we are forced to lift our skirts or present a bloodstained sheet to prove our virginity, the fact remains: There is only one first time. There is no perfect age for sexual intercourse, and although we may experience pressure from our partners, our peers, or the media, it has been proven that it is better being older rather than younger before we engage in sexual intercourse. Teenage depression and attempted suicide are three times more prevalent among teenagers who are sexually active, and two thirds of teenagers report that they wish that they had waited longer before becoming sexually active.

Before we indulge in sexual intercourse and share the beauteous secrets that our lady-love-lies possess, we need to ask ourselves a few questions:

- Is it legal? (Am I older than sixteen?)

- Do I actually *want* to have sex?

- Does it fit into my personal belief system (family, cultural, and religious orientation)?

- Am I in a loving relationship with healthy and open communication?

- Do I know enough about my partner, pregnancy, contraception, and sexually transmitted diseases?

- Will I be pleased when I look back later in life with the way in which, and with whom, I lost my virginity?

If you're not yet ready to go down this road of unreserved sexual intimacy, certainly refrain from using alcohol to numb the warning signs. You should rather indulge in passionate and fulfilling sexual expressions like hugging, kissing, and massaging. Although the urgency to gratify our innermost desires may be overwhelming, do take great care to make informed decisions regarding this momentous event.

CHAPTER 8

THE EFFECTS OF SEX
ON THE VAGINA

Although coitus is our congenial vehicle to reproduction, sexual intercourse is often performed exclusively for pleasure and as an expression of love and emotional intimacy within a relationship. Have you ever wondered what happens to our vaginas before, during, and after having sex?

The sexual response has four stages: excitement (arousal), plateau, orgasm, and resolution, and all of these stages can also be experienced during masturbation, manual stimulation by one's partner, or oral sex. During the excitement phase, which is signaled by vaginal lubrication, the vagina becomes longer and wider, the clitoris enlarges, the labia swell and separate, and the uterus rises slightly.

The plateau phase marks the zenith of sexual excitement before orgasm and may be achieved, lost, and regained several times without the occurrence of an orgasm. During this phase, the vagina and labia continue to lubricate and swell; the uterus tips to position itself high in the abdomen and, as the orgasmic platform develops, the lower part of the vaginal opening also swells, narrows, and tightens.

During the orgasmic phase, the sexual tension that has been building in the body is diffused and endorphins, which cause a sense of unparalleled well-being, are released. Orgasm may involve spasms and a heavenly loss of awareness for those fortunate ones among us, or it may be indicated by as little as a sigh of subtle relaxation. During this time of euphoria, the vagina, the anus, and the muscles of the pelvic floor contract five to twelve times at 0.8-second intervals.

Resolution is the period following orgasm during which the muscles relax and the body begins to return to its pre-excitement state. The clitoris shrinks slightly and resumes its prearousal position, the labia return to normal size, the vagina relaxes, and the cervix opens to help semen travel up into the uterus. Around twenty to thirty minutes after an orgasm, the cervix closes

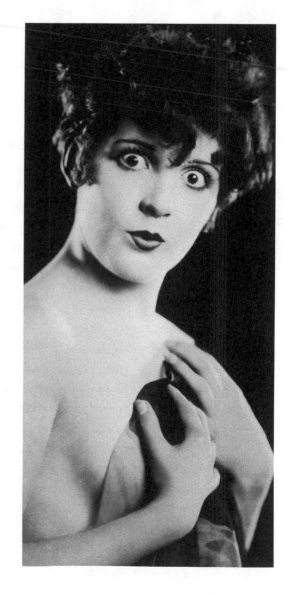

this highway to heaven, and the uterus lowers into the upper vagina. Our bodies are, beyond doubt, amazing in their responses during our interlude of shared pleasure.

THE HISTORY OF CONTRACEPTION

Since there is a host of easily obtainable information on modern contraception, let us take a quick look into the history of birth control—even if it is for no other reason than to appreciate our luck at having been born later rather than sooner. Some of the earlier methods are archaic and somewhat bizarre, and you will be well advised *not* to try them at home.

The Greek, Soranus of Ephesus (early second century AD), the greatest gynecologist of antiquity, advised women to hold their breath and draw the body back during sex so that the sperm could not penetrate the mouth of the uterus. To dislodge the sperm, he prescribed jumping backward seven times after intercourse. Ancient Rome had its own prescriptions for contraception: Some women wore a leather pouch containing a cat's liver on their left foot during sex, others carried a lucky charm of mule earwax, and—my personal favorite—still others practiced prevention by spitting three times into the mouth of a frog. Women were also encouraged to turn the wheel of a grain mill backward four times at midnight or to insert a finger into the vagina and gently swirl it around to dislodge and "confuse" the sperm.

In an ancient medical manuscript, the Ebers Papyrus (1550 BC), our fellow Eves were advised to grind dates, acacia tree bark, and honey into a paste and apply it to the vulva with seed wool, which is cotton wool not yet cleansed of seeds. Other concoctions that were applied around the vagina included mixtures of olive oil, pomegranate pulp, ginger, and tobacco juice. The use of pessaries (vaginal suppositories or diaphragms) appears as early as the second century BC. The Kahun Papyrus (1850 BC) promotes vaginal plugs of crocodile dung and fermented dough as guaranteed sperm barriers. Other plugs contained cocoa butter, boric and tannic acid, apricot stones, honey, tree gum, and bark. Softer options included inserting objects such as sea sponges or soft wool soaked in either lemon juice or vinegar. For a spur-of-the-moment sexual rendezvous, half a lemon was inserted into the vagina.

The Arabs were the first to place pebbles strategically into the uteruses of their camels so that they remained "unhindered" during long trips through the desert. This marks the first use of intrauterine devices in the history of contraception. German physicians Carl Hollweg (1902) and Richard Richter (1909) were the first to insert pessaries into their patients' uteruses, and Ernst Gräfenberg, the previously mentioned gynecologist who discovered the G-spot, first reported the clinical performance of an intrauterine device (IUD) made from silkworm gut and wire coiled into a ring. This method proved to be very effective (it had a 3 percent pregnancy rate in 1928, and the following year that percentage dropped as low as 1.6 percent) and is still very popular today.

Oral contraceptives have been used for more than four thousand years. Options ranged from drinking urine and eating animal and plant parts to sipping poisons such as arsenic,

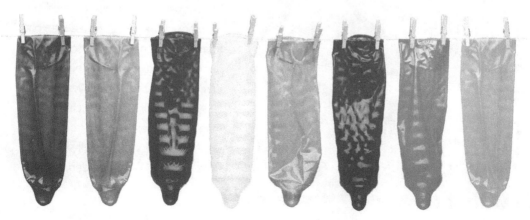

mercury, and strychnine. While women in India enjoyed eating carrot seeds, an aboriginal group in Eastern Canada imbibed tea brewed with beaver testicles. Unquestionably, that's not everybody's cup of tea!

In prehistoric times "penis protectors" were used to safeguard men from insect bites, evil spirits, and injuries; to ornament the body; to promote virility; or to indicate rank. Only later was the protector used as a contraceptive barrier. Then it was manufactured from animal bladders or intestines, which evolved into linen condoms devised by the Italian physician, Gabriello Fallopius in 1564. Fallopius had a 100 percent success rate with these in the prevention of syphilis. The famed seducer Giacomo Casanova (1725–1798) reportedly fashioned these fine linen "glans hoods," which only covered the tip of the penis. They were soaked in a chemical solution, allowed to dry, and quaintly tied to the penis with a ribbon.

Throughout the ages, glans condoms were made from oiled silk paper, tortoise shell, and animal horn. The earliest rubber condoms also covered only the glans of the penis, and a doctor had to measure each man's erect penis in order to supply a custom-fit hoodie. The name *condom* possibly derives from the Persian *kendu* or *kondu,* which means "a long storage vessel made from animal skin." The world's oldest, full-sized condom, found in Lund, Sweden, is made

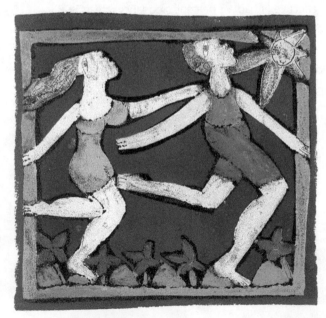

Leslie Xuereb, *Summer Love*

from pig intestine and dates back to 1640. This model was reusable and issued with a user's manual, written in Latin, with instructions to immerse the condom in warm milk prior to use to avoid diseases.

A condom is the only contraceptive aid that is effective in both birth control and in the prevention of sexually transmitted diseases. This little roll-up device is also our most trustworthy ally in our quest to fight the deadly AIDS pandemic. It is relatively inexpensive, reliable, light, compact, and disposable, and it requires no medical supervision and has no side effects. Nowadays, condoms are made from latex or polyurethane. Polyurethane condoms are mostly recommended when a woman or a man has an allergic reaction to latex. They are more costly than the latex varieties, but they are also thinner and apparently more pleasing in texture and appearance.

Contraceptives today include a selection of birth control devices, pills, spermicides, implants, and injections, and this is not to mention the full range of condoms of diverse textures, shapes, sizes, and colors, including the female variety. Designer condoms, which promise to take one's sexual bliss to the next level, include an assortment of glow-in-the-dark, flavored, studded, ribbed, spiral-shaped, scented, and lubricated types. Be thankful that you can decline sipping beaver testicle tea, turning the mill at midnight, or be challenged, in your moment of ardor, by a man with a horn on the tip of his penis!

However, there does come a time when we deliberately throw caution to the wind in an attempt to become pregnant. According to the Minnesota State University Museum, pregnancy testing in ancient times included urinating on planted emmer and barley seeds. If the barley grew, it would be a boy; if the emmer sprouted, it would be a girl. If neither grew, the woman was clearly not pregnant.

CHAPTER 9

PREGNANCY AND CHILDBIRTH

The miracle of pregnancy is universal and timeless, and even though we are, by divine design, capable of going through this process, it does have a pronounced effect on our bodies and our sexuality. During this event, higher levels of progesterone cause drowsiness while the increased estrogen lifts our mood, making us more radiant than ever. As our bodies gradually grow larger, we may suffer from stormy hormonal changes. Suddenly we have irrepressible cravings and our sense of smell becomes acute; we have whimsical shifts in preferences and aversions, and if exposed to the sun, we may even acquire a pigmented "moustache" and brown patches on our cheeks.

During the fourth month of pregnancy, our vaginas become puffy and enlarged, and the color of the labia deepens considerably. Both the increased blood supply to the vagina and the increased pressure on it create a permanent state of gentle sexual arousal, leaving us moist and more conscious of our lady parts. The thin line that runs between our pubic patch to our navels also becomes more pronounced.

As far as childbirth goes, we have a number of options: We can have our babies come into this world via our vaginas or our abdomens. Both methods have their fair share of health benefits and burdens, and your health practitioner will be able to assist you best in making the right choice for both you and your baby.

Childbirth may seem like a daunting task; thoughts of bright lights and a narrow trolley bed, and us with our legs raised and splayed, leave us feeling exposed and vulnerable. Furthermore, our breasts blow up like balloons, and it seems we leak from all of our orifices.

The possibility of suffering a vaginal tear or having to have an episiotomy during natural vaginal birth is an equally scary

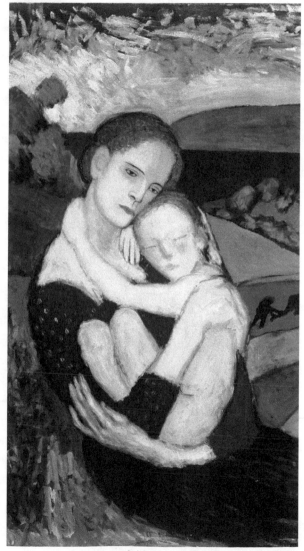

Pablo Picasso, *Motherhood (La Maternité)*

thought. (An episiotomy is an incision made from the base of the vagina toward the anus to enlarge the vagina and assist in childbirth.) Note that after an episiotomy the female's perineum is stitched up; the stitches in the perineum, which are tight and prickly, must stay in for approximately two weeks after the birth. Sheila Kitzinger advises that one can press a witch hazel–soaked sanitary pad against these stitches while emptying the bladder to alleviate pain and discomfort, and once the stitches have dissolved, gently massage the area with arnica oil and direct a warm stream of air from a hair dryer to aid the healing process. It's no wonder we often feel bruised, battered, alienated, fragile, and invaded after giving birth to our babies. Needless to say, we begin to wonder if we'll ever be the same again.

The good news is that the discomfort and state of despair soon abate to allow for sentiments of a more mystical, sensual, and serene nature: Feelings of awe gently seep into our frame of mind as we realize the miracle of this extraordinary experience. This leaves us feeling delicately feminine, yet strong and empowered.

Soon after childbirth, hormonal levels return to their pre-pregnancy levels, except in breastfeeding moms, for whom it will take longer as they continue to have high levels of prolactin and oxytocin in their systems throughout the lactating stage. About 80 to 90 percent of women resume intercourse three months after delivery, but nearly 70 percent of new mothers experience sexual dysfunction. This does not come as a surprise. Mentally we may be ready to engage in intimate pleasures, but our body's response lags behind. Sexual problems after giving birth relate to decreased libido, difficulty in achieving an orgasm, vaginal dryness, and *dyspareunia*. Dyspareunia is painful sexual intercourse due to physical or psychological causes. All we need during this recovery phase is a little TLC and patience (and perhaps a lubricant) as these complaints typically resolve themselves during the first year after childbirth.

The most common long-term problems associated with childbirth include urinary incontinence and pelvic organ prolapse. Although incontinence (the "laugh-and-leak" syndrome) and prolapse (sagging of the organs) are dealt with in more detail in Chapter 10, we do need to look at pelvic-floor function since injury in this department is closely, but not exclusively, related to pregnancy and childbirth.

The pelvic floor consists of a complex, multilayered group of muscles, tissues, and nerve endings that creates a hammock between the pubic bone and the base of our spinal cord and supports a number of organs including the bladder, rectum, uterus, urethra, vagina, and anus. The pelvic floor seems to be the "headmistress" that has all our lady parts neatly secured in her firm hand. She has the huge task of coordinating, directing, and protecting all of our beneath-the-belt bits, and she plays a valuable role in our womanly health. We should be well aware of her strengths and shortcomings.

Apart from pregnancy and childbirth, other factors such as smoking, a weak genetic disposition, spinal cord injuries, chronic coughing and constipation, a hysterectomy, hormone replacement therapy, menopause, aging, and excess body weight can have negative impacts on the function of the pelvic floor.

During pregnancy, however, the weight of the baby, the "water," and the placenta put a twenty-times-heavier-than-normal strain on the pelvic floor, and this often leads to urinary incontinence during the last trimester. Vacuum extraction, forceps delivery, an episiotomy, lying on the back, and applying fundal pressure (pressing on the abdomen to help move the baby out) are all factors that increase pelvic injury risk during vaginal birth. Even by opting for a caesarean section we are not exempted from pelvic injury risk; in fact, this procedure inceases the risk of maternal death by sixteen-fold, and it increases the risk of having to have a hysterectomy by ten times.

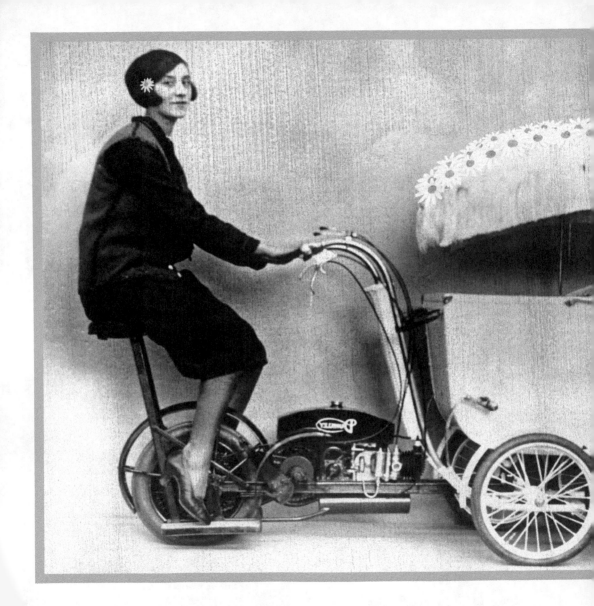

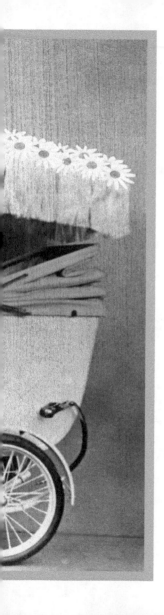

The best and safest way to protect ourselves from pelvic-floor impairment is Kegel exercises. The importance of these exercises cannot be overemphasized; they play a vital role in the prevention and treatment of pelvic-floor disorders. Work those muscles daily to keep them strong, elastic, and toned. 🖝

CHAPTER 10

A CHANGE OF SEASON

Pills, reading glasses, walking sticks, sagging breasts, arthritis, thinning hair, wrinkles, and liver spots.... In *A Companion to Ethics*, Gerald Larue reminds us of the delightful "Epic of Gilgamesh." Gilgamesh, the king of Uruk (2700 BC) was a demigod credited with possessing superhuman strength. He was obsessed with immortality and spent all of his energy finding ways to evade death. His travels took him to one of his forefathers, Utnapishtim, who had been granted eternal life by the gods. Utnapishtim instructed Gilgamesh, who fervently hoped to receive the same gift, to forfeit sleep for six days and seven nights to attain immortality. But, needless to say, the mere mortal fell asleep. Utnapishtim then offered Gilgamesh eternal youth, a gift hidden in a plant at the bottom of the ocean. Gilgamesh successfully retrieved the plant, but while he was resting, a snake slithered by and devoured the magic plant. And there you have it! Not only are we predestined to die, but, unlike the snake that can shed its old, dried-out skin to appear eternally youthful, we have no prospects for rejuvenation. Aging is our fate, and so are pills, reading glasses, walking sticks, sagging breasts....

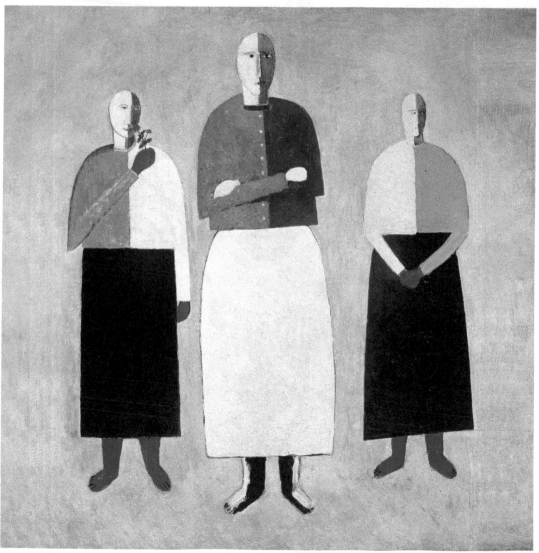

Kasimir Malevich, *Three Girls*

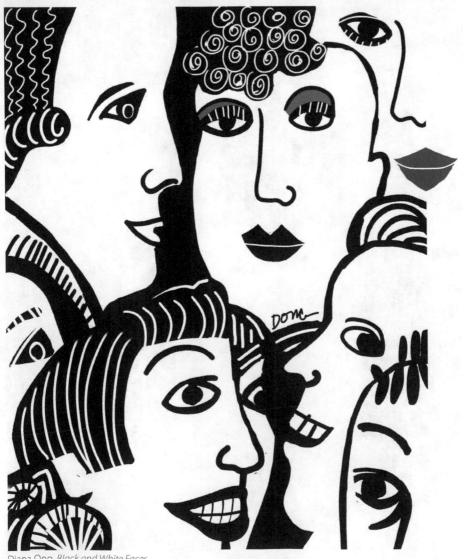

Diana Ong, *Black and White Faces*

As if aging is not enough, menopause hits us with hot flashes, night sweats, insomnia, bladder and urinary-tract problems, heart palpitations, headaches, fatigue, mood changes, and general irritability. It certainly is not true that change is as good as a holiday. Moreover, it is decidedly untrue that we have to surrender to feelings of doom and gloom; as with everything in life, the more informed we are, the better equipped we will be to embrace new beginnings.

HOW DOES THE COOKIE CRUMBLE AS WE GET WISER?

Change is inevitable as we grow older, and, apart from becoming wiser, more content, comfortable, confident, and stronger on both emotional and spiritual levels, our bodies, too, will signal a number of changes. This transition period, when our menstrual cycle comes to a halt, is also called the climacteric and occurs over the course of a few years. Although 8 percent of women are menopausal before the age of forty, the "pause" normally sets in around the age of fifty.

The term *climacteric* is not used exclusively in relation to women; it also refers to the midlife crisis that men experience around the same time. Certainly we are not alone during this time of change; male menopause sufferers report many symptoms similar to their female counterparts such as irritability and other negative moods, muscle and joint aches, depression, sleeplessness, fatigue, and headaches. Although most men are seemingly only slightly affected by these symptoms, some climacteric men are easily spotted: They have a bronzed, overly tanned appearance, often complemented by a white baseball cap that covers the thinning hair on the shiny crowns of their heads. These gentlemen usually sport tasseled leather loafers and a diamond-encrusted Rolex and drive a shiny convertible that is considered by many people to be the classic "male menopause vehicle" (MMV)!

But let us remain focused on the changes under our own belts.

We can expect thinning, balding, or graying of our wild and woollies. As the "bush" clears, the vulva becomes more pronounced. This should not cause alarm since we have already learned to love our own "dark continent"; allow her to step unashamedly into the limelight. And then there are, of course, many ways to color and cut our curlies, but more about that in Part III, in which we discuss hair care down there.

Our little love button, now fashioned with more character (yes, wrinkles!), appears larger as the fold of skin that covers the clitoris shrinks and retracts. Although the clitoris may become highly sensitive, even too sensitive, it gives us no reason to catnap in this department. One of the best remedies for menopause and aging is to make use of our lady lovelies more often. The increased blood flow to the vagina from sex counters dryness, and by maintaining the sizzle in our sex lives we can burn calories, gain energy, sleep better, reduce headaches and joint pains, strengthen our immune system, improve our cardiovascular health, and slow down the aging process.

The outer arena of our most intimate crevice, the vulva, also shows signs of aging: It appears less distinct since the connective tissues and fatty deposits under the skin start shrinking. The first change takes place under the pad of fatty tissue covered by the pubic hair (the mons pubis). This part is lovingly referred to in some countries as the "Beetle bonnet" (from Beetle, the VW car, and "bonnet," which is referenced to as a car's "hood" in the United States). Not unlike all models of motor vehicles, which change shape over time, we too can fashion a more sporting look. Furthermore, we can also expect the lips of the vagina (the labia) to become less plump, more pendulous, and frilly.

These symptoms correlate with a condition called vaginal atrophy (degeneration); it occurs in 15 percent of premenopausal women and in 10 to 40 percent of postmenopausal women. Vaginal atrophy, in addition, causes the walls of the vagina to become narrower, shorter, less elastic, and considerably thinner. The vaginal opening, meanwhile, becomes smaller. Thinning mucous membranes may result in chronic irritation such as dryness, itching, burning and general discomfort. A dry vagina carries an increased risk of infection, and penile penetration can cause small tears, ulceration, bleeding, and, again, infection. A topical, twice-weekly application of estrogen cream effectively combats vaginal atrophy. Vaginal secretions, now more watery, become less frequent. Higher pH levels may also occur when our vaginas become atrophic; the normal level of between 3.8 and 4.5 may rise to between 6.0 and 7.5, which further adds oil to the infection fire. For more information on infections, refer to Part IV.

Lastly, the muscles, ligaments, and other tissues that support the pelvic floor, bladder, uterus, vagina, and rectum will lose their tautness, resulting in possible organ prolapse. Vaginal prolapse occurs when the front and back walls of the vagina become weakened and begin to move downward and literally slip out of place. Look out for swelling around the opening of the vagina, or bulges at the back, inside wall.

Bladder prolapse, a condition that occurs in 37 percent of women, unkindly bequeaths us with leaking when we laugh, sneeze, or exercise. When we suffer from incontinence (the involuntary loss of urinary control caused by bladder prolapse), we may experience a feeling of pelvic pressure or fullness, have difficulty when urinating, or encounter painful uterine contractions.

CROSSING THE BRIDGE

Given this rather negative and myopic view of the changes we can expect "down under," we are naturally inclined to feel defeated and pessimistic. It is, nevertheless, unnecessary to be left high and dry—let us restore our poise and self-confidence with the following valuable solutions.

Vaginal Dryness

To counteract a dry vagina, women should make adequate lubrication part of their playtime routine, as it will help with painful intercourse. Water-based lubricants, such as K-Y Jelly, are safe to use and are easily obtainable over the counter. Stay away from oil-based, "spray-and-cook" gimmicks and petroleum products such as Vaseline. These are not only tricky to flush out of the vagina but may also perpetuate irritation or infection. Furthermore, these products may cause the disintegration of latex condoms. Taking vitamin E, enjoying foods rich in essential fatty acids, and drinking enough water are also effective actions to take in combating vaginal dryness.

A topical estrogen preparation can be applied in and around the vagina. It relieves the dryness and enhances the appearance, thickness of the skin, and pH levels. Some of these life-saving creams are, in low dosage, available over the counter, but the more concentrated products are available only by prescription. As the estrogen cream is absorbed through the skin, it may cause side effects, so it should therefore be applied only in small quantities. Consult your doctor if you experience any adverse effects that may include dizziness, heartburn, vomiting, double vision, irritability, sensitive nipples, or muscle and joint pains.

Hormone replacement therapy (HRT), which entails the systemic replenishment of estrogen, or combinations of estrogen and other hormones such as progesterone, is also helpful in countering vaginal dryness. Let your medical doctor's close observation and support guide you along this route, which is too complicated and specific to address within the scope of this book.

Vaginal Prolapse

Kegel exercises should faithfully be incorporated into our regime to prevent our kit and caboodle from slipping out of place. Multivitamins, if taken regularly, are also known to be beneficial in the prevention of organ prolapse: Vitamins A and C help with the formation of collagen, and the mineral manganese helps to maintain healthy bones, cartilage, and skin. In more severe cases, a nonsurgical treatment is available. This entails inserting a pessary, a small plastic cone holding a tiny weight, into the vagina to strengthen and support the pelvic-floor muscles.

In serious cases of prolapse, surgery, either abdominal or by means of a laparoscope (via the navel), is recommended. Approximately 11 percent of women will undergo this procedure by the age of eighty, and 30 percent of these will have to repeat the surgery due to recurring symptoms. A surgical repair can last twenty to thirty years, and success is, to a large degree, guaranteed if we are at our ideal weight and if we have this operation before entering menopause, as we have more collagen and estrogen premenopausally, which will aid the healing process.

When we are, as a result of bladder prolapse, burdened with incontinence, options include the insertion of vaginal pessaries or repositioning the bladder surgically. The latter is done by inserting a sling or by raising and securing the urethra to the surrounding muscles, ligaments, or bones. The sling, made from a synthetic-mesh material or the patient's own tissue, is placed under the urethra to substitute the deficient pelvic-floor muscles and provide a hammock of support.

A PAUSE FOR THOUGHT

Female sexuality is surrounded by myths, taboos, and personal beliefs. One such fallacy is that women lose interest in sexual activity after menopause, but aging and sexual dysfunction are not inexorably linked. Even though our genital engorgement during the excitement phase does take longer (fifteen minutes or more as opposed to five minutes in our younger years) and is less intense, it only means that we need a little more foreplay. And the good news is that time

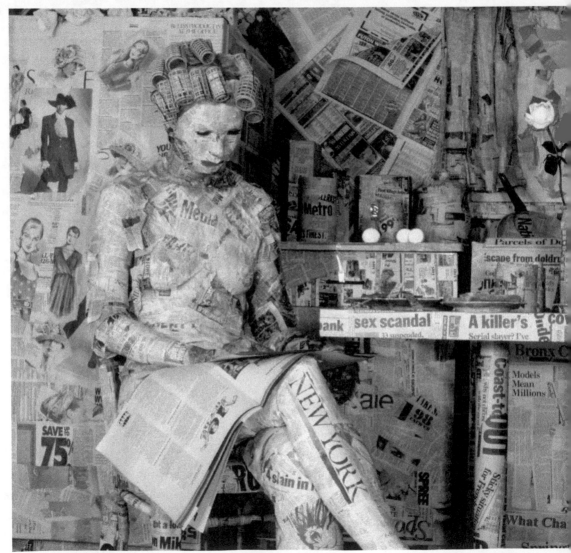

Filippo ioco, *Read Me*

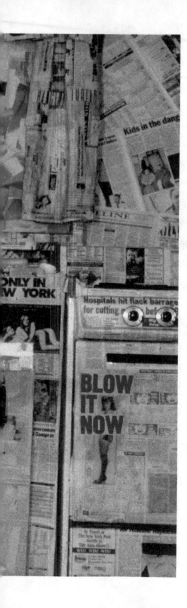

is a luxury we do enjoy in our golden years. Women who remain sexually active throughout the years are less affected by delayed lubrication than their celibate counterparts. Furthermore, vaginal atrophy is significantly less prevalent among women who have intercourse more than three times per week than among those who have intercourse less than ten times per year.

The plateau phase of sexual response is also prolonged in older women, which suggests that we can take pleasure in the heavenly bliss of preclimax excitement for a little while longer. It is good to know that, according to a study in the *Western Journal of Medicine* (1997), 56 percent of women over the age of 60 years continue to be sexually active, and that 74 percent of these women enjoy intimacy at least once a week.

Even *more* impressive is the fact that 30 percent of women between the ages 80 and 102 continue to be sexually intimate with their partners. Sexual inactivity in older women is largely due to loss or illness of a partner or their inability to "rise to the occasion." Among women who remain sexually active, 94 percent derive emotional fulfillment and 91 percent receive physical satisfaction from their relationships. Postmenopausal women not only enjoy a strong libido; some say they also enjoy improved sex in their autumn years! Up to 82 percent of women who take HRT and 69 percent of women not taking

HRT claim that their sex lives have remained unchanged or have improved during and after menopause. And while 54 percent of women report that they think about sex more frequently while on HRT than they did ten years before, 34 percent state that their present sexual desire is as strong as it was in their thirties.

Postmenopausal women celebrate having more everyday fun and greater independence, and they say that they feel more content and in control of their lives. Contributing factors in achieving a positive, postmenopausal life include good nutrition, exercise, plenty of rest and sleep, a greater overall balance in life, fewer child-rearing responsibilities, increased job satisfaction, and meaningful relationships with loved ones. Regular exercise has a beneficial effect on hot flashes, joint pains and aches, overall well-being, body mass index, and the risk of coronary heart disease. It improves our vitality, mental health, and overall quality of life.

Factors that speed up the onset of menopause are smoking and malnutrition. Typically, women who smoke reach menopause two years earlier than nonsmokers, and under- or malnourished women begin the process of menopause up to four years earlier than women who are well nourished. It is evident that lifestyle and social circumstances influence health-related quality of life more than the menopausal transition stages as we grow older. In our graceful amble beyond menopause and toward our golden years, it is important to view all changes as natural, exciting, and fulfilling enhancements of our lives. We will live one third to half of our lives after menopause, so we might as well embrace this time and make the most of it. To call this a period of crisis is debatable. Perhaps, more accurately, it is our hour of happy hiatus, a time to catch our breath.

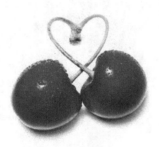

Old age is far more than white hair, wrinkles,
the feeling that it is too late and the game finished,
that the stage belongs to the rising generations.
The true evil is not the weakening of the body,
but the indifference of the soul.
— André Maurois, 1885–1967

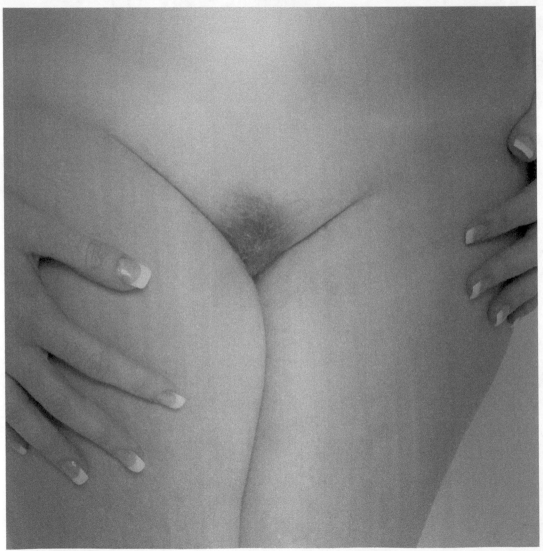

Milan Cronje, *Ginger*

PART III

COOKIE COIFFURE: GROOMING OUR SHORT AND CURLIES

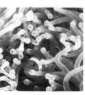

CHAPTER 11

TATTOOING AND BODY PIERCING

Body adornment in the form of tattoos and piercing has been practiced for many centuries. The word *tattoo*, meaning "to mark something," comes from the Tahitian word *ta-tau*, which mimics the sound of a little wooden hammer as it taps a small needle, dipped in ink, under the skin. In April 1769 Captain James Cook, on his second journey to the South Pacific, discovered a group of islands called Tahiti, and, with it, the art of ta-tau. Omai, a colorfully tattooed, indigenous Tahitian, joined Cook on his return journey and his appearance sparked off an enthusiasm for skin decoration among British royalty. This marks the introduction of tattoos to the Western world.

The practice of tattooing has been a tradition with many cultural groups around the world and has served as a rite of passage, markings of fertility, symbols of religious and spiritual devotion, and decorations for bravery, sexual lure, and pledges of love. In addition, tattooing has also been used as marks of punishment to ostracize outcasts, slaves, and convicts and even as an identification system for concentration camp inmates during the Holocaust. Today, however, people choose to "color in" for cosmetic, erotic, sentimental, military, and religious reasons; to show devotion to a particular individual; or to display affiliation with a particular subculture.

Vaginal tattoos are normally placed on the mons pubis and can continue up onto the stomach or down onto the upper, inner thigh to "frame" the genital area. Tattoo aficionados may even incorporate the hair to create an overall look, like a bird's nest or a beard, for instance. Since the tattooing of the inner labia poses a serious risk of infection, decorative needle art is normally restricted to the outer skin regions.

If one is lured into treating the body as a canvas, it is probably best to experiment with a henna tattoo—an ancient practice that allows artistic freedom without pain or permanence. Many centuries ago, the henna plant was used medicinally for the treatment of jaundice, leprosy, smallpox, skin complaints, sore joints, thrush, flatulence, and burns. The most common association with

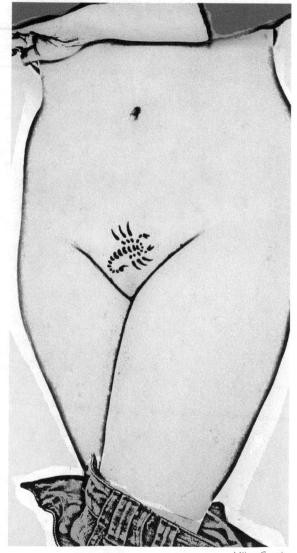

Milan Cronje

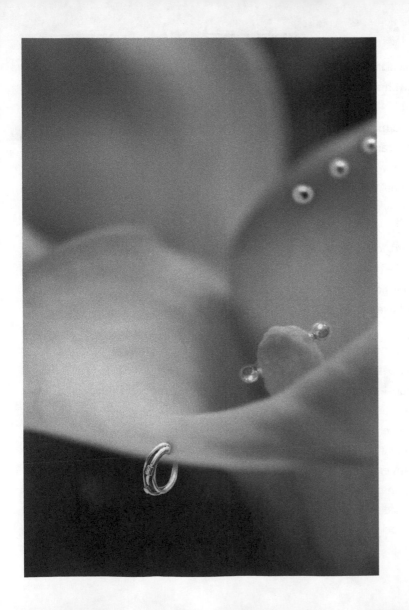

henna tattooing is its use within the Indian culture as a ceremonial art form for wedding cere-monies. The leaves of the henna plant are ground into a powder, mixed into a paste, and applied to the skin, resulting in a reddish brown stain. Only a small percentage of women are allergic to henna, which leaves the invitation open to most of us to experiment with these eye-catching tattoos. A henna tattoo lasts for up to two months and is available in a vast range of attractive designs that can be used for special occasions.

Body piercing has an even longer history that tattooing. The oldest mummified body, Ötzi the Iceman (c. 3300 BC), was found to flaunt an ear piercing, ⅓ to ½ inch in diameter. Julius Caesar (c. 100–44 BC) introduced earrings as a male status symbol, and in the Elizabethan period, many men, including William Shakespeare, Sir Walter Raleigh, and Sir Francis Drake, are known to have worn them.

Caesar's elite centurions wore nipple rings as a sign of their virility and courage, and na-vel piercing served as a symbol of royalty among the ancient Egyptians. In typical tribal fash-ion, we find that the Amazonian tribal hunters and gatherers still display bullrings to intimidate their prey and appear more fearsome. Women of the Matsés tribe in the Amazon rain forest are likewise decorated with ornaments in their noses to represent the whiskers of cats; hence the name, the "Cat People."

More specifically, however, we'll take a look at the bells and whistles of genital piercing. The "Prince Albert," named after the beloved husband of Queen Victoria, is probably the most doc-umented and recognized example of a "down-there" piercing. Whether this "dressing ring" was originally used to secure the penis to either the right or the left leg to visually diminish a man's natural endowment during the Victorian craze for extremely tight, crotch-trussing trousers remains unclear. This piercing, usually a circular or curved barbell, goes through the head of the penis and the frenulum, which is the elastic band of tissue under the glans of the penis.

"PrinceAlbert" devotees claim that it makes the penis aesthetically more attractive and provides greater stimulation for both partners during sex.

For women, a fair choice of genital piercing locations is offered. The clitoral hood seems to be the most preferred piercing site and is alleged to enhance both vaginal pleasure and outward appearance. It has the fastest healing period, and rings, studs, or barbells can be used to penetrate this fleshy fold either horizontally or vertically. Next follows the labia minora, which can be pierced multiple times to form a decorative line on the soft inner fringes.

A more painful piercing with a slower healing period, undertaken only by the most devoted of piercing enthusiasts, can be performed on the labia majora. The latest addition to the genital piercing fashion is the "Fourchette," in which a captive bead ring or curved barbell is placed through the base of the vaginal opening into the perineal tissue. Although the rejection rate is high for this newcomer, it is not a very painful procedure, and healing occurs quite rapidly.

Before we decide to beautify our vaginas with genital jewelry, we must be aware of the possible health hazards that this practice poses. Piercing carries an increased risk of viral infections like hepatitis B, hepatitis C, and the human immunodeficiency virus (HIV). Bacterial infections, although seldom serious, do affect 10 to 20 percent of pierced poonannies.

Allergic reactions are usually caused by nickel genital jewelry—it is therefore best to use high-quality ornaments manufactured from titanium or niobium. Lastly, excess scar tissue that leads to the formation of a keloid may also result from improper piercing methods, careless hygiene, or overstretching of the skin. Women who are predisposed to keloid formation should be extra cautious.

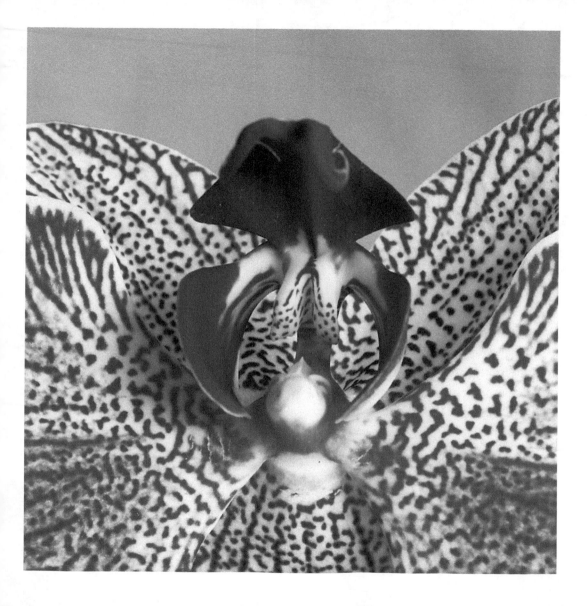

CHAPTER 12

COLOR, CUT, AND CURL

According to Dr. Terry Hamilton, the Chinese refer to pubic hair using poetic terms such as "black rose," "fragrant grass," "sacred hair," or "moss." They also draw an entertaining and refreshing comparison between personality and the texture or color of pubic hair: If your fur is black and bushy, it indicates that you are a strong and obstinate woman; a brown love-mound with golden tints is indicative of being easygoing and generous; and short, fine, and silky hair tells us that you are quiet and introverted. Furthermore, it appears the more bountiful and bushy you are, the more passionate and sensual your nature, and if you are fortunate enough to have growth forming a trail of hair right up to you navel, you are considered truly beautiful!

Pubic hair keeps us warm, protects our sensitive lady parts from external friction during intercourse, collects secreted pheromones, and serves as a visual indicator of sexual maturity. There are an number of reasons, however, why we choose to shave, pluck, wax, electrolisize, or lazer our wild and woolies. Some of these may include having pubic lice, fleas, or other parasites; in preparation for surgery; or for religious, cultural, or sexual reasons. Lastly, we may delight in pubic grooming for matters relating to aesthetics and creative, personal expression; British fashion designer Mary Quant (b. 1934) was famously proud that her husband trimmed her pubic hair into a heart shape.

In Western art, female nudes were unrealistically portrayed as being smooth and hairless for many a year: We find the first depiction of pubic hair in *La Maja Desnuda*, a painting by the Spanish master Francisco de Goya, which hangs in the Museo del Prado, Madrid. This earlier misrepresentation had the famous nineteenth-century British author, artist, and art critic John Ruskin at a loss for words on his wedding night. When he discovered that his lovely wife, Effie Gray, had a thatch of hair down there, he thought that she was freakish and malformed. Their marriage, which was never consummated, was annulled six years later.

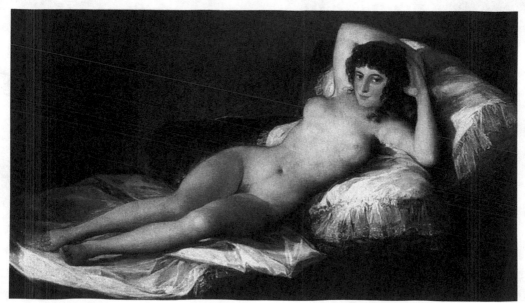

Francisco de Goya, *La Maja Desnuda*

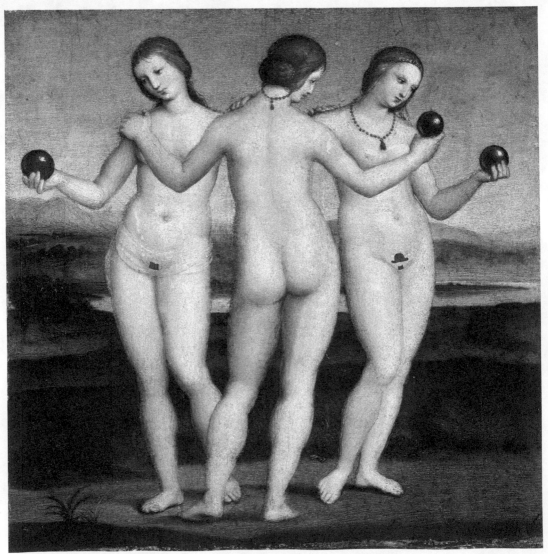

Milan Cronje, *Raphael's Three Graces inspired by Charlie Chaplin*

Today we are more daring and public about pubic matters. So, ladies, let us be brave and bold (or bald, if you so wish!) and indulge in trendy ways to comb, cut, color, and condition our warm and beautiful fuzzies. We can draw our inspiration from nature or comedy or exploit special occasions to set the stage. Let us try it out for a season, perhaps for no reason, or purely for a laugh! This personal expression of our private selves, albeit a little *risqué* and naughty in a really nice way, holds some wonderful promise. Apart from enhancing our sensuality, it simply makes us feel fabulously feminine.

We'll start with the classics. The "bikini cut" is the most conventional form of tidying up our bushy business. Here we remove only the straggly bits so that no hair is visible when we don our underwear or bathing suits. A more daring expression of this style is the "Faux '70s" look, where we keep it full but trimmed on top and smoothly shaven between our legs, exposing the puffy, flowery bits of our vaginas.

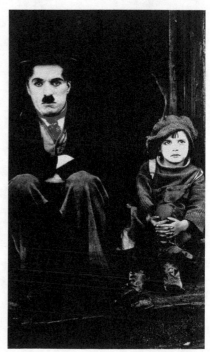

Then there is the well-known "landing strip," which leaves a straight path of hair on the mons veneris, or a narrower version of the same style, the "Brazilian." The origin of the Brazilian dates back to a letter written by Pêro Vaz de Caminha (1550 AD) documenting Pedro Álvares Cabral's voyage to Brazil, which translates: "their private parts were so exposed, so healthy and so hairless, that looking upon them we felt no shame."

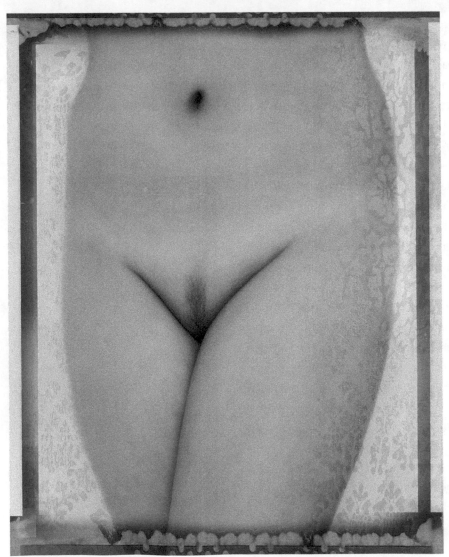

Milan Cronje, *Classic Landing Strip*

It leaves us with the "Hollywood," which is also known as "The Sphinx." This name derives from the smooth-skinned, hairless Sphinx cat that is a genetic oddity first bred in Toronto in 1966. With this cut, all the curlies are removed, leaving the genitals completely exposed.

Some women may be alarmed that men who express an interest in smooth-skinned, hairless pussycats may be secretly harboring a desire for underage girls, but apparently quite the opposite is true. Males are instantly aroused by the fully matured anatomy that is so confidently and openly displayed. On the next two pages are a few more furry, fun ideas...

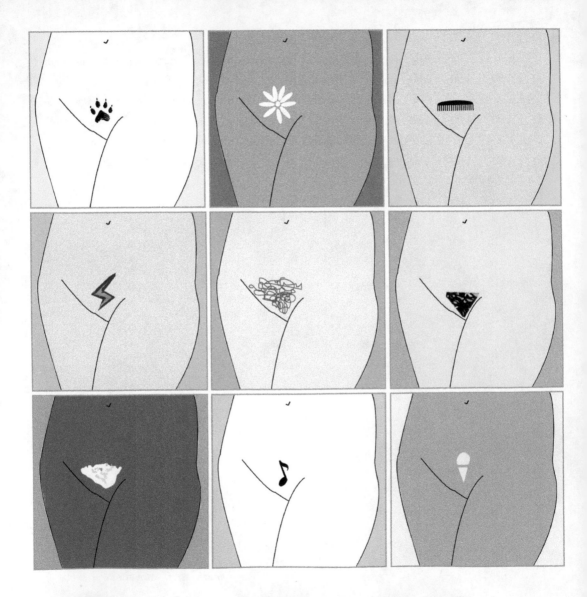

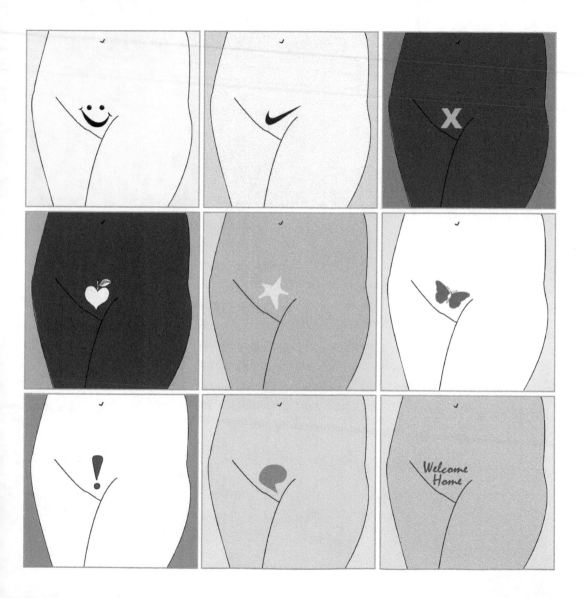

CHAPTER 13

HAIR CARE DOWN THERE

There are many methods to temporarily or permanently remove pubic hair, and this can be discussed with your specialist beautician. Nevertheless, the biggest problem that we do experience with hair removal is the itchy regrowth and the incidence of ingrown hair.

We've all had to deal with those annoying, itchy, and tender red bumps at some time or another. But again, there is no reason why these indecorous dots should put the brakes on our creative expression. *Pseudofolliculitis barbae* is the correct term for ingrown hair, and it occurs when the hair curls back into the skin instead of growing *through* the skin, which then causes irritation, inflammation, or infection of the hair follicles. Luckily, *Pseudofolliculitis barbae* is a condition that can quite easily be prevented or treated.

PREVENTING INGROWN HAIR

First, if our curlies are wild and unruly, we should trim them before we shave, as this will prevent our razors from clogging up with hair. Use a pair of scissors or an electric shaver but be careful.

We don't want to snip anything but hair! After that, employ a gentle scrub, using a loofah or a "puff," to remove dead skin in preparation for a smoother shave. A gentle scrub is the best way to prevent ingrown hair, and the practice should be maintained between shaving and/or waxing sessions.

It is best to wait a little before we shave. The steam and heat from the shower will open the pores slightly and soften the hair. It is crucial to use a clean, sharp, good-quality razor; blunt blades are a definite no-no. Apply a mild, hypo-allergenic shaving cream with a moisturizer for sensitive skin and leave it on for a minute or two. Again, both the hair and the skin will soften, making it easier to shave.

Second, when shaving, refrain from applying too much pressure, shave *with* the grain to avoid skin irritation, and don't shave repeatedly over the same area. Cleanse the area with

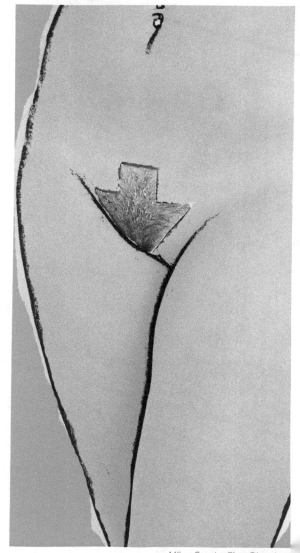

Milan Cronje, *Clear Direction*

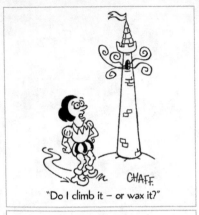

"Do I climb it – or wax it?"

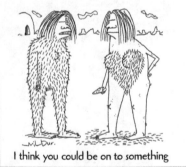

I think you could be on to something

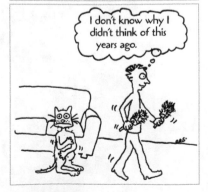

a gentle, antibacterial soap (a facial product for sensitive skin also works well) and lightly pat dry. You can apply an unscented, vitamin E–rich moisturizer, but again, be vigilant. We want to moisturize only the outer skin, so stay away from the sensitive inner-labia region. Last, but not least, wear cotton underwear and avoid tight-fitting garments that may cause unnecessary friction and irritation.

TREATING INGROWN HAIR

Refrain from hair removal and don't scratch any itchy patches until the condition has cleared up. To take care of the red bumps, a topical anti-inflammatory cream is helpful, and in severe cases a small amount of cortisone cream can be applied. If you have an infection, which is identified by little white heads on the red bumps, use a natural antiseptic agent such as tea tree oil. If the condition doesn't clear up after a few days, it's best to see your doctor.

You could also gently try to extract the ingrown hair from the follicle. Have a long bath or shower to open the pores slightly and loosen and soften the hair. Use sterilized tweezers to carefully manipulate the rebel until it is loosened and then remove it from the follicle. There are also products on the market for ingrown hair that you can obtain from your pharmacist or from your beauty specialist. These will not only prevent ingrown hair but will also be helpful in treating the condition.

And don't forget home remedies; they may take a little longer to clear up the condition, but they are well worth trying. Salt has exfoliating qualities, increases circulation, promotes healing, and reduces swelling. One also might soak in a warm bath with two cups of Epsom salts or apply salt directly to the wet skin and work it in with gentle, circular motions.

Sugar is another wonderfully mild scrub that will leave the skin silky and smooth. One cup of sugar can be mixed with ½ cup of extra virgin olive or jojoba oil to moisturize the skin and make it easier for the hair to push through the surface. In addition, ten drops of both tea-tree and lavender essential oils can be added to the sugar mixture; the former has antiseptic properties, and lavender oil combats inflammation and redness. Gently work the scrub using circular motions on wet skin and then rinse it off. The remaining sugar scrub can be stored in an airtight container. Use it daily if you suffer from redness and irritation or, alternatively, apply it twice a week to prevent red spots.

Finally, use an aspirin mask for itchy, red dots. Aspirin contains salicylic acid, which has powerful exfoliating properties and fights inflammation. But before you dive into your first aid kit, consider one warning: *Do not* use this remedy if you are pregnant, breastfeeding, allergic or sensitive to aspirin or salicylic acid, or have any medical condition that prohibits you from taking aspirin.

Here is the mask recipe. Simply crush three or four uncoated aspirin tablets, mix with ½ teaspoon of water or Jojoba oil, and add 1 teaspoon of honey. Mix the ingredients in a small bowl, and then place the bowl in a bigger basin filled with hot water to allow the mixture to soften. If you have oily skin, aspirin can be mixed with water alone; otherwise, jojoba oil can be added to moisturize dry skin. Honey can also be mixed into this concoction as it possesses natural hydrating, antiseptic, and antibacterial properties. The temperature of the mask should be pleasantly lukewarm as you spread it over the ingrown hair with your fingers; after ten minutes, rinse your face with warm water and pat dry. An aspirin mask once or twice a week should be enough to counter even severe inflammation and redness. One final warning: After you have had a wax treatment, wait for a few days before applying an aspirin mask, and do not use one if your skin is cut or sunburned.

Now that we have scrubbed, sugared, and spiced until we are satin soft and well groomed, let's drop in and say a quick hello to the vagina's next door neighbor — the anus (Latin: *ānus*, which means "ring"). A squeaky-clean anus will help prevent vaginal infections and an itchy bottom, so here's the trick. Dab a few drops of baby oil onto a tissue and gently wipe, front to back, over the anus. This will remove all traces of stool residue and leave you with a healthy "ring around the rosy."

We have covered pubic grooming and hygiene, but the question of anal bleaching remains. We all have some degree of skin pigmentation on or around the anus. This can be mistaken for poor personal hygiene or viewed as aesthetically unappealing, possibly fuelling an interest in anal bleaching. There are a number of products available to lighten the skin in this region, but many, if not all, of these products contain harmful chemicals such as hydroquinone. Hydroquinone is a chemical substance banned in many countries. Its corrosive properties may destroy or irreversibly damage the skin and subcutaneous tissue, leaving one particularly vulnerable to contracting sexually transmitted diseases (STDs) and HIV. Side effects include scarring and anal burning, and it may even cause an inability to pass stools. These darker-as-we-grow-older outer layers of tissue come with the territory and are vital in protecting the anus and the vagina, and it is, beyond a shadow of a doubt, dangerous to bleach this area.

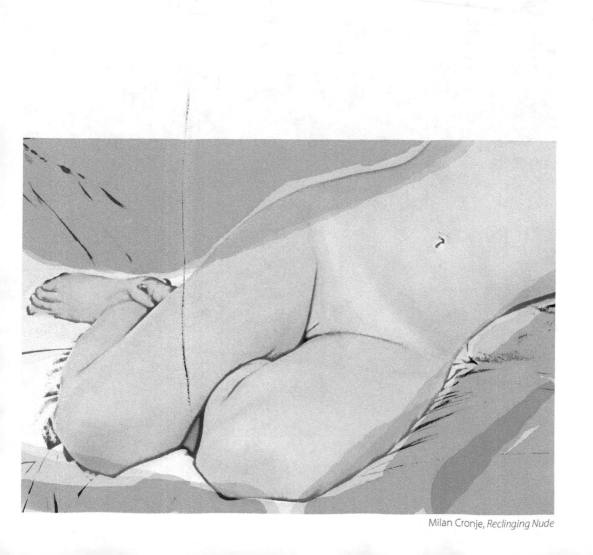

Milan Cronje, *Reclinging Nude*

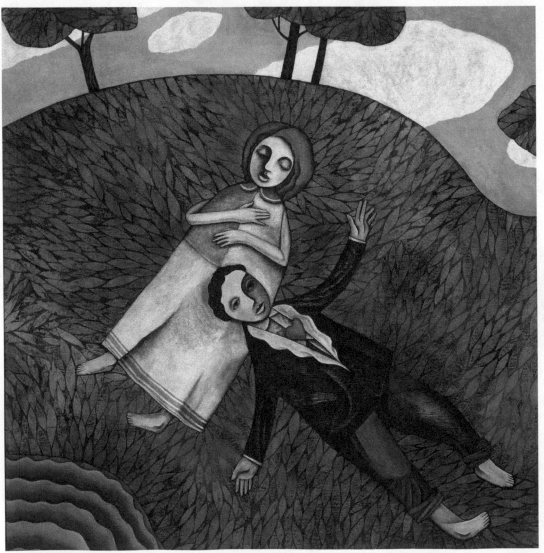

Daniel Nevins, *River Diego*

PART IV

FEMME FRESH: MEDICAL MATTERS

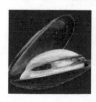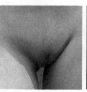

CHAPTER 14

THE WANDERING UTERUS

When it comes to the health of women, our forefathers had some strange ideas. "Hysteria," a condition attributed solely to women, was, according to the Egyptian Kahun Papyrus (c. 1900 BC), caused by an alleged "wandering uterus." This upward migration of the uterus had women "aching in all their limbs with pain to the sockets of their eyes." The Greeks espoused this idea; it was progressively recognized throughout the Middle Ages, and the notion remained popular during the European Renaissance of the fourteenth to seventeenth centuries. Richard Mead (1637–1754), one of the most successful English physicians of his time, stated that there was "no disease so vexatious" as hysteria.

Diseases of Women, the authoritative gynecological treatise of Hippocrates (c. 460–370 BC), offers a comprehensive account of this "terrifying" condition. It states that a woman's womb becomes heated, light, and empty from hard work, which then causes it to turn and rush up into the moist belly. As the womb turns, it collides with the liver, which causes sudden suffocation, and "she turns up the whites of her eyes and becomes chilled; some [become] livid. She grinds

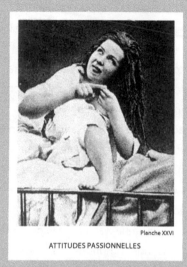

Planche XXVI

ATTITUDES PASSIONNELLES

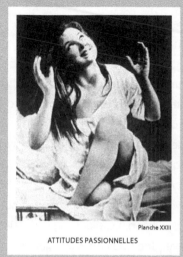

Planche XXIII

ATTITUDES PASSIONNELLES

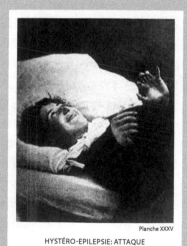

Planche XXXV

HYSTÉRO-EPILEPSIE: ATTAQUE

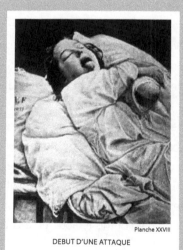

Planche XXVIII

DEBUT D'UNE ATTAQUE

Hysterics under hypnosis, *Iconographie photographique de la Salpêtrière (Paris, 1877–1880)*

her teeth and saliva flows from her mouth: if the womb lingers near the liver and the abdomen, the woman dies of suffocation."

Two treatments were developed to combat this condition. Either a sweet-smelling, vaginal fumigation was used to lure the uterus back into its original position, or foul-smelling substances, such as animal dung and urine, were inhaled or ingested to repel the uterus away from the upper cavities to where it had "wandered." Vaginal fumigation allowed for vapors to be admitted by means of a hollow, perforated, artificial penis that the woman inserted before squatting over a smoldering fire. Vaginal pessaries made with opium poppies were also used. Furthermore, the area below the liver was pushed down and a bandage tied below the ribs while strongly scented wine was poured into the patient's mouth.

During the Middle Ages (500–1400 AD), hysteria was such a widely recognized problem that even the Church became involved. The "wandering uterus" was addressed in much the same way as the devil, and chants such as the following were recited to heal the tormented lady: "I conjure you, womb, by our Lord Jesus Christ, who walked on the waters with dry feet, by whose bruises we are healed. By Him, I conjure you not to harm this maidservant of God, not to hold onto her head, neck, throat, chest, ankles, feet or toes, but to quietly remain in the place God delegated to you, so that this handmaiden of God may be cured."

According to Rachel Maines, virgins were encouraged during the Victorian era to marry healthy, virile men and to have sexual intercourse frequently, as this was believed to "discipline" the disobedient and obstinate uterus. For those who were single, horseback riding and bouncing enthusiastically in a swing were considered helpful. If all else failed, one last option remained: the direct, manual stimulation of the genitalia until a "hysterical paroxysm" was reached. A "hysterical paroxysm" [**parr**ok-sizm] is an intense orgasm induced by a medical practitioner. Doctors soon tired of this tedious, time-consuming task that could last anywhere from four minutes to an hour. Midwives were employed to assist until a medical device, the first clockwork powered vibrator, the "trémoussoir," was invented in 1734. This very expensive medical instrument was exclusively used in asylums and by the medical profession to curb hysteria.

Another form of treatment, the "hydratic pelvic massage," became a favorite after the first spa that offered this therapy opened in 1760 in Pennsylvania. In the middle of the nineteenth century, hundreds of similar spas were established in America and Europe. These so-called "pelvic douches," which aimed a strong stream of water at a lady's exterior pelvic area, were a very effective orgasm-inducing tool. They alleviated hysteria in just four minutes!

In 1869 George Taylor created a steam-powered vibrator, the "Manipulator," which was superseded by the electromechanical vibrator in 1883. In 1899 a battery-operated appliance became available that was sold directly to the consumer. Oddly enough, the occurrence of "wandering uterus hysteria" sharply declined during the early twentieth century and seems to have disappeared since. Thanks should also be given to the work of Jean-Martin Charcot and Sigmund Freud in the late nineteenth century who, due to a greater understanding of and a more scientific approach to psychological matters, reclassified hysteria into a more definable neurosis.

Hopefully, your uterus is sufficiently disciplined and not given to roaming. Now, without further ado, let us return to the twenty-first century and the medical marvels that now help remedy our sometimes unhappy vaginas.

CHAPTER 15

VAGINAL INFECTIONS

Vaginal discharge, or so-called love juices or *aqua vitae* (the "waters of life"), is a normal and natural element of a healthy vagina. It does not smell unpleasant and is not accompanied by pain, itching, burning, or redness. The amount of discharge is just enough to moisten the vaginal opening and may leave a light yellow stain on undergarments when it dries.

Normal vaginal discharge varies with age, our menstrual cycle, sexual arousal, pregnancy, and the use of birth control routines or other hormone replacement medication. Teenage girls, for instance, may have excessive amounts of watery discharge caused by high hormonal levels. Our aqua vitae also thickens, increases, and becomes slightly gluey when we ovulate. This creates a welcoming environment for contending sperm racing up through the uterus. Preperiod discharge normally has a brownish or deep-red hue, and its appearance constitutes the first day of menstruation.

Vaginal discharge during pregnancy is more abundant, sometimes whitish in color, quite sticky, and a little thicker than normal. This is a normal consequence of high levels of estrogen

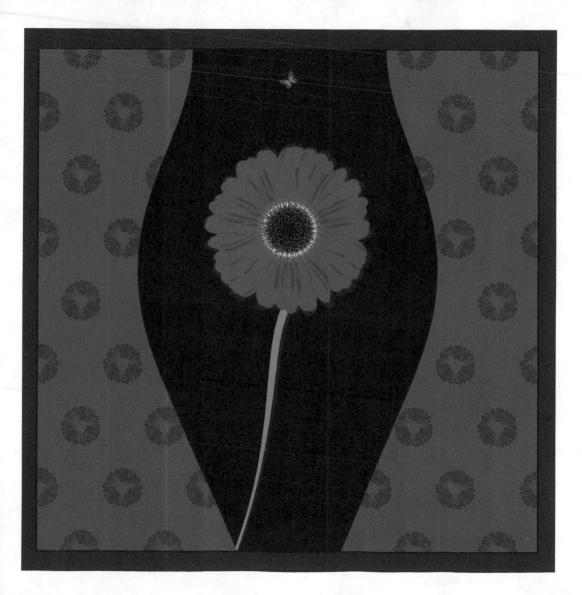

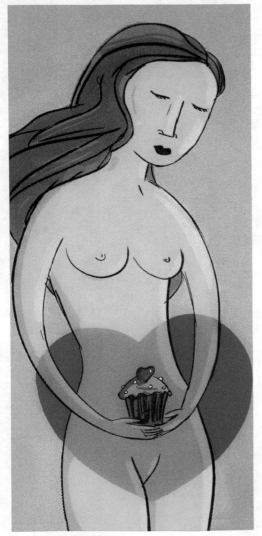

David Kuijers, *Cupcake*

and progesterone. Because of Mom's high hormonal levels, her unborn baby girl's genitals are also stimulated during pregnancy. This results in a vaginal discharge in all newborn baby girls — secretions that soon disappear as the estrogen levels wear off.

Our vaginal discharge serves as a good indicator of our intimate well-being, as changes could be signaling that all is not well down south. An offensive-smelling discharge may be a warning of vaginal infections, an infection of the cervix, foreign objects in the vagina, or a sexually transmitted disease.

The three most common types of vaginal infections are yeast infections, bacterial infections, and trichomoniasis, which is a parasitic infection. Vaginitis (inflammation of the vagina) is caused by these infections, all of which can be treated with oral or vaginal preparations.

There are also a number of preventative measures that we can take to reduce the occurrence of vaginal infections:

- Use condoms during sexual intercourse.

- Switch over to a polyurethane variety if allergic to latex condoms.

- Do not douche unless it is prescribed by a medical practitioner.

- Wear only cotton underwear; nylon and lycra don't allow for sufficient moisture absorption.

- Sleep without panties.

- Refrain from wearing too-tight garments.

- Be naughty and expose your vagina for a few minutes to direct sunlight and fresh air — apart from making you feel sexy, it is also healthy.

- Do not use perfumed soaps, scented tampons and sanitary pads, or intimate deodorants or sprays.

- Use only white, unscented toilet paper.

- Keep the anus super clean and prevent contamination by wiping front to back.

- Limit bubble baths to special occasions.

- Change out of wet bathing suits as soon as possible.

- Drink alkaline powder and enough water to assist with general well-being and maintaining a balanced pH level.

- Drink cranberry juice; it has antibacterial properties and helps maintain a healthy bladder.

- Take pleasure in a healthy lifestyle, which includes a diet with lots of fresh fruit and vegetables.

- Apply plain yogurt to the vagina when you have slight burning and irritation.

- When traveling abroad, take your own tampons from home to reduce the risk of developing toxic shock syndrome. Toxic shock syndrome (TSS) is a rare but potentially fatal illness caused by a bacterial toxin that is linked to some high-absorbency tampons.

- Change tampons regularly (never leave one in for longer than eight hours) and avoid the use of tampons to protect against incontinence leaks.

- Use a water-based lubricant such as K-Y Jelly if you experience vaginal dryness.

- If you find you are sensitive to or allergic to certain detergents and fabric softeners, find ones that don't irritate you, such as those without added fragrance.

- Don't scratch if you experience itchiness; it perpetuates irritation.

VAGINAL YEAST INFECTION

Candidiasis [cande-**di**-asis], thrush, or yeast infection, is very common; three out of four women suffer from this fungal infection. It occurs when we have an excess growth of yeast organisms in the vagina that causes itching, swelling, and sometimes pain during urination and intercourse. It produces a thick, white discharge from the vagina, much like cottage cheese. Although symptoms are inconvenient and annoying, thrush rarely leads to serious problems.

Factors such as antibiotics, oral contraceptives, hormone replacement therapy, douching, pregnancy, tight-fitting clothes, a weakened immune system, diabetes, obesity, and large amounts of sugar, starch, and yeast in the diet, can increase the risk of developing a vaginal yeast infection. It sometimes comes and goes without medication, but if it persists, antifungal creams and vaginal suppositories are obtainable over the counter without a doctor's prescription.

BACTERIAL VAGINOSIS

Bacterial vaginosis (BV), also known as nonspecific vaginitis, results from an imbalance in the normal bacterial flora of the vagina. It's good to have a healthy mix of bacteria in the vagina, but when antibiotics or a pH imbalance, for instance, allow more resistant bacteria to gain a foothold, it produces a thin, yellow or grayish, foul-smelling ("fishy," if you like) discharge that is accompanied by itching, burning, and inflammation. Bacterial vaginosis is very common; one in three women will have to deal with it at some point in time. It most commonly presents itself in sexually active women between the ages of fifteen and forty-four years, with higher incidences in pregnant or menopausal women, women under stress or in woman-to-woman sexual contact. Thongs are also said to be notorious for causing bacterial vaginosis due to the fabric rubbing against the anus and the vagina. In prepubescent girls, bacterial vaginosis may be caused by bacteria introduced from the anus owing to improper hygiene after bowel movements, or by the chafing effect of underwear and tight-fitting garments.

Although this infection is mostly viewed as a mere nuisance, untreated bacterial vaginosis may cause pelvic inflammatory disease (PID), an increased susceptibility to sexually transmitted infections, and premature births of infected babies. BV is treated with antibiotics in the form of creams, gels, or tablets as prescribed by one's medical doctor. Precautionary actions include using tea tree products designed for application around the vagina, using condoms, and taking probiotic tablets orally.

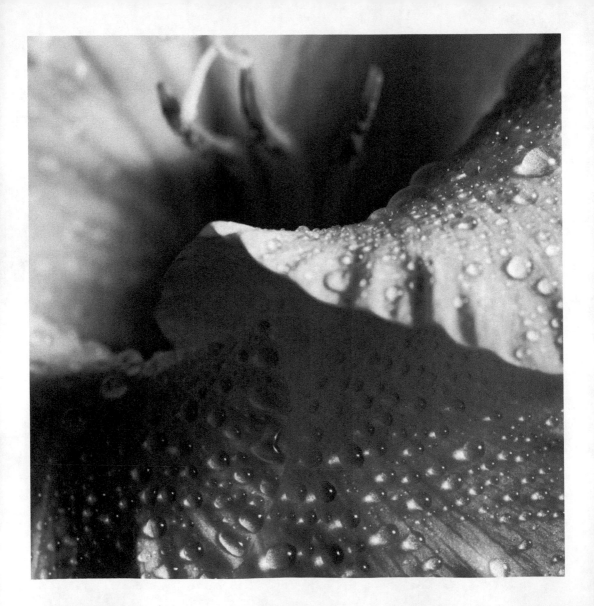

TRICHOMONIASIS

Trichomoniasis [trick-o-mo-**nai**-sis] or "trich" is a common cause of vaginitis, and one can become infected by sharing external water sources like a Jacuzzi, using wet bathing suits and towels, or engaging in sexual intercourse. It is considered the most common nonviral sexually transmitted disease. The telltale signs are burning, itching, and discomfort during or after intercourse and urination, and a frothy, yellow-green vaginal discharge, usually with a strong smell.

The trichomonad is a microscopic parasite that can be dormant for years, but symptoms appear when the body's natural defense is swamped by a large number of reproducing trichomonads. Although "trich" is more annoying than dangerous, research shows that it increases the risk of HIV transmission and that it may be responsible for low birth-weight or premature deliveries of newborn babies. Trichomoniasis is easily diagnosed with a quick trip to your medical doctor, who will prescribe an antibiotic treatment.

FOREIGN OBJECTS

If your vaginal valley produces a green discharge, accompanied by an unpleasant odor, you need to dig a little deeper as the most likely cause is a foreign object like a tampon or a birth control device forgotten in the vagina. These girly tools should come with forget-me-not instructions!

Before you pursue the task at hand, wash your hands with soap and water, squat down or sit on the toilet, or stand and put one foot on the bathtub. Use two fingers and sweep them back and forth inside your vagina to try and detect the string attached to the object. Gently tighten your lower abdominal muscles as if you are going to have a bowel movement, and push to lower the object down into the vagina. Once your feel the string or the object, grasp it firmly and remove. After a successful attempt, you will have immediate relief; if you are unable to locate anything, be brave and hand the task over to your health professional.

EXCESSIVE OR ABNORMAL VAGINAL BLEEDING

When you consult your doctor regarding abnormal bleeding, you'll most likely be asked about your cycle, so it is wise to keep a record of your periods—it will also provide you with a good indication of your own, unique biological rhythm. "Spotting" refers to light bleeding between menstrual periods, and may be caused by oral contraceptives, hormone fluctuations, or intrauterine contraceptive devices.

Menorrhagia [men-o-ray-**jee**-a], on the other hand, is a condition that occurs in about 10 percent of women and refers to excessively heavy menstrual bleeding. Normally, women lose less than a ¼ cup of menstrual fluid per month, which results in ten to fifteen soaked tampons or pads. Excessive bleeding can be caused by a number of reasons. Commonly, it results from hormonal imbalances triggered by the use of oral contraceptives or by problems with the thyroid, ovaries, pituitary, or adrenal glands. A miscarriage or complications during pregnancy may also cause abnormal bleeding, as will cysts, scars, and other growths on the cervix or uterus. Injury to the vagina during sexual assault or surgery or the presence of foreign objects may also be responsible for excessive bleeding. Other culprits include sexually transmitted diseases or endometriosis.

Endometriosis is a condition in which tissue similar to the lining of the uterus (which should only be located inside the uterus) is found elsewhere in the body. These cells can invade the ovaries, the Fallopian tubes, the vagina, the bladder, the skin, and even the lungs, spine, or brain. Invasive and excessive growth can distort a woman's internal anatomy and literally fuse the internal organs together. An estimated 30 to 40 percent of women with endometriosis may not be able to have children. The most common symptom of endometriosis is pelvic pain, which should be treated and managed with the help of a medical doctor.

Off-cycle bleeding is a natural element of the perimenopausal phase, which indicates the gradual onset of menopause. This phase can last between four and ten years, and symptoms include irregular menstruation, mood changes, hot flashes, and vaginal dryness. However, postmenopausal women who experience bleeding should immediately consult a doctor since benign or cancerous tumors of the ovaries or uterus are a probable cause. Excessive bleeding accompanied by fever, abdominal pain, or unusual mucus or other substances emitting from the vagina may indicate an infection that should be treated by a medical practitioner.

Isn't it unfortunate that the incalculable treasure of being a woman is weighed down by such an infinite list of things that can go wrong? But then, this balance between divinity and vulnerability does make us truly human.

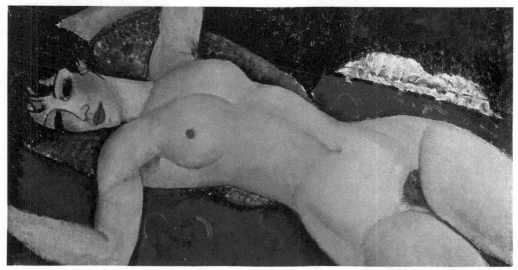

Amedeo Modigliani, *Red Nude*

CHAPTER 16

SEXUALLY TRANSMITTED DISEASES

Sexually transmitted diseases (STDs) are infections that are transferred from one person to another through any form of sexual contact. Sexual contact includes oral–genital contact, the use of sex toys such as vibrators, and even kissing. Although condoms are useful in preventing the spread of certain infections, they do not fully protect us against genital herpes, genital warts, or syphilis. Furthermore, although many STDs are treatable, vaccines are not yet available to effectively remedy them all.

Unfortunately, the unequivocal truth is that "safe sex" hardly exists. If we want to luxuriate in the ceremonies of harmless pleasure, we really have only two options: either abstain or be in a long-term, monogamous relationship in which both partners have been tested and neither is infected with an STD. Casual lovers, or infected partners, may literally love us to death.

The most common STDs, apart from "trich," are gonorrhea, chlamydia, syphilis, genital herpes, human papillomavirus, chancroid, ectoparasitic infections, and HIV.

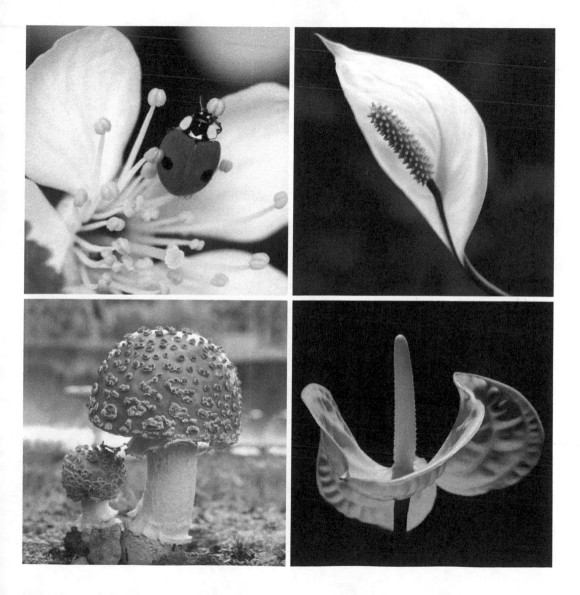

GONORRHOEA

Gonorrhoea [gone-o-**ree**-a] is a sexually transmitted disease and, contrary to popular belief, cannot be transmitted via toilet seats. The bacterium *Neisseria gonorrhoeae* can live outside the body for only a few seconds or perhaps for a minute or two, at most. These bacteria grow and multiply effortlessly in the warm, moist areas of the reproductive tract and can also grow in the mouth, throat, eyes, and anus.

Although any sexually active person can be infected with gonorrhea, the highest reported instances are among sexually active teenagers and young adults. Once infected, many women show no early stage symptoms but, in due time, the faithful companions of infection such as burning and frequent urination, a yellowish discharge, and redness, swelling, burning, and itching of the vaginal area will follow.

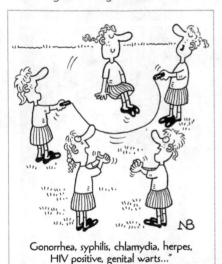

Gonorrhea, syphilis, chlamydia, herpes, HIV positive, genital warts..."

A doctor can confirm gonorrhea by taking a swab of the infected site, after which both partners will be treated with a single or multiple dosage of penicillin or quinolone. If left untreated, gonorrhea leads to severe pelvic infection accompanied by inflammation of the ovaries and Fallopian tubes. Our ovaries, or reproductive organs, are situated on each side of the uterus (womb), and secrete our female hormones and produce eggs (ova).

The Fallopian tubes are two thin, flexible muscular structures that connect the ovaries with the uterus and provide a passageway for the eggs to travel to the uterus. It is also here in the Fallopian tubes where conception—the fertilization of an egg by a sperm—normally takes place. Babies who pass through an infected birth canal can suffer from blindness, joint infection, or a life-threatening blood infection, or they can be stillborn.

Condoms are effective in protecting us from gonorrhea but since the organism can live in the throat, condoms should be used during oral–genital contact as well.

CHLAMYDIA

Chlamydia [cla-**me**-deea] is a bacterium that is very similar to gonorrhea in the way it spreads and in the symptoms that it produces. It can be transmitted during vaginal, anal, or oral sex. Often a woman is unaware of this infection until she starts suffering from cervicitis, which is the most common manifestation of the infection. Cervicitis is an infection of the cervix, which is the lower region of the upside-down, pear-shaped womb (the uterus) that projects into the vagina. The cervix has a small opening, only big enough to allow fluids to pass through. During childbirth this opening widens sufficiently to allow for the baby to be delivered vaginally.

Some women may have symptoms such as excessive discharge, abdominal pain, or an urgent and frequent need to urinate. If untreated, chlamydia can cause pelvic inflammatory disease (PID), leaving us infertile, as it is very harmful to the Fallopian tubes.

Premature births are associated with this infection, and babies too can become infected with this bacterium during their passage through a contaminated birth canal, leading to serious eye damage or pneumonia. Because of these potential threats, all newborns are treated with eye drops containing an antibiotic that kills chlamydia.

Chlamydia can be detected by swabbing the cervix during a conventional examination or, alternatively, one can have a urine sample tested, which is less invasive. Treatment involves antibiotics and, as with gonorrhea, a condom, used for vaginal and oral sex, prevents the spread of the infection.

SYPHILIS

Syphilis [**sif**-a-lis] is caused by a microscopic bacterium. The wormlike, spiral-shaped organism wriggles when viewed under a microscope, burrows into the moist, mucus-covered lining of the mouth or genitals, and produces a painless ulcer known as a chancre [**shang**-ker].

Syphilis is known to have three stages, and the first two are highly contagious. Stage one produces an ulcer on the outside of the vagina or in the mouth, which means that an innocent kiss can infect us. Although the chancre will heal without treatment after three to six weeks, it is imperative that this stage is treated to prevent the secondary and tertiary stages from developing.

Secondary syphilis is the systemic stage of the disease, which means that it attacks various organs of the body. The most common development is a nonitchy, highly contagious skin rash that typically appears on the palms of the hands or the bottoms of the feet. Other symptoms include hair loss, sore throat, fever, headaches, wartlike lesions on the genitals, and white patches in the nose, mouth, and vagina.

A latent phase, which can last for ten to twenty years, is followed by the tertiary stage of the disease. Although no longer transmittable, this stage causes a range of problems that can be fatal: heart problems, strokes, mental confusion, meningitis, sight deterioration, deafness — and in the case of pregnancy, blindness, delayed development, or even death in infants may occur.

People who suffer from syphilis have an estimated two- to five-fold increased risk of contracting HIV. Syphilis can effectively be treated with penicillin or other antibiotics. Condom use can reduce the risk of potential exposure but only if the infected area is covered. Any unusual discharge, abscess, or rash, particularly in the groin area, signals a need for an immediate trip to the doctor.

GENITAL HERPES

Genital herpes [**hur**-peez] is a highly contagious virus that has the ability to cast its appalling shadow permanently on our systems. It enters the lining of our vaginas or our mouths through microscopic tears and travels up to the nerve roots near the spinal cord and settles there forever. Outbreaks, in the form of redness and blisters, reoccur whenever our immune systems are suppressed or stressed by other infections or medication.

There are two types of herpes viruses: herpes simplex virus-1 (HSV-1) and herpes simplex virus-2 (HSV-2). HSV-1 is generally responsible for blisters in and around the mouth while HSV-2

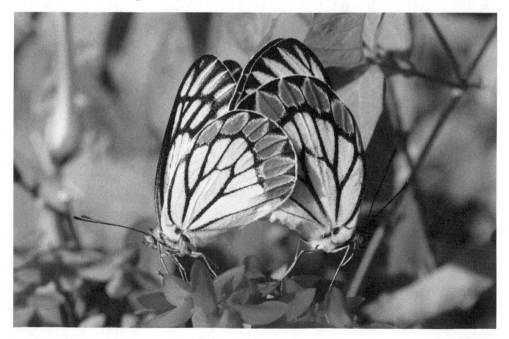

causes genital sores or lesions in the area around the anus and vagina. Up to 60 percent of sexually active adults carry the herpes virus. Some are unaware of the symptoms as atypical outbreaks are accompanied only by mild itching and minimal discomfort. Typical outbreaks cause a tingling sensation followed by redness and blisters that are very painful to touch. This virus can be transmitted even in the absence of a recognizable outbreak.

Although there is no known cure for herpes, there are antiviral treatments that will alleviate and reduce the severity and duration of outbreaks. Treatment, as recommended by your doctor, should be started as soon as the familiar, pre-outbreak tingling sensation occurs or at the very onset of blister formation. During this time all sexual contact, including kissing, should be avoided.

HUMAN PAPILLOMAVIRUSES AND GENITAL WARTS

There are more than forty types of human papillomaviruses [pap-a-**low**-ma-viruses], which cause genital warts, cervical cancer, and cancer of the genitals and anus. The human papillomavirus (HPV) is considered to be the most common sexually transmitted infection; at least 75 percent of the reproductive-age population has been infected at some point in their lives.

Genital warts are small and fleshy and may form flat, stalklike trails or appear as cauliflower or ticklike bumps. Warts aren't painful but are sometimes associated with itching, burning, or tenderness. These unwelcome growths often form clusters in and around the vagina, in the cervix and the uterus, and around the anus. Although asymptomatic carriers of a HPV have no conspicuous warts, they are still able to spread the infection through sexual contact.

People who have many sexual partners, as well as those who have had unprotected sex, are most vulnerable to this infection. Anyone in doubt should consult a doctor for a clinical examination. It is advisable to go for regular Pap smears to screen for cervical cancer and pre-cancerous changes in the cervix. A Pap smear, which is named after its inventor, Georgios Papanikolaou (1883–1962), is a quick and painless procedure in which your doctor gently cleans your cervix with a cotton swab and then collects a sample of cells that is sent to a laboratory to be examined. If you have had several episodes of a yeast infection, you should also consider being tested for HPVs, as chronic yeast infections make a woman more vulnerable to STDs.

Apart from removing the warts, which unfortunately doesn't guarantee that regrowth will not occur, there is no cure or treatment that will eradicate an HPV infection. Condoms also prove to be ineffective in preventing the spread of this resilient infection.

Nevertheless, there is some good news: A recent medical breakthrough offers two vaccines that can protect us from these viruses. Cervarix prevents HPV types 16 and 18, and Gardasil protects us against types 6, 11, 16, and 18. These vaccines are safe to use and prevent cervical cancer, precancerous lesions, and genital warts.

The vaccines prove most effective for boys and girls between the ages of nine and twenty-six years—especially those who have not already been exposed to HPV. Some of us have missed this opportunity, but for those who are still in this window, an ounce of prevention is most certainly worth a pound of cure. Let us encourage our children to be vaccinated; this is definitely a shot all young women should take!

CHANCROID

Chancroid [**shang**-croid] is caused by a bacterium that produces a tender bump on the penis, the outer surface surrounding the vagina, or the inner thighs. After some time, this tender bump will swell, burst, and become a painful open sore (ulcer).

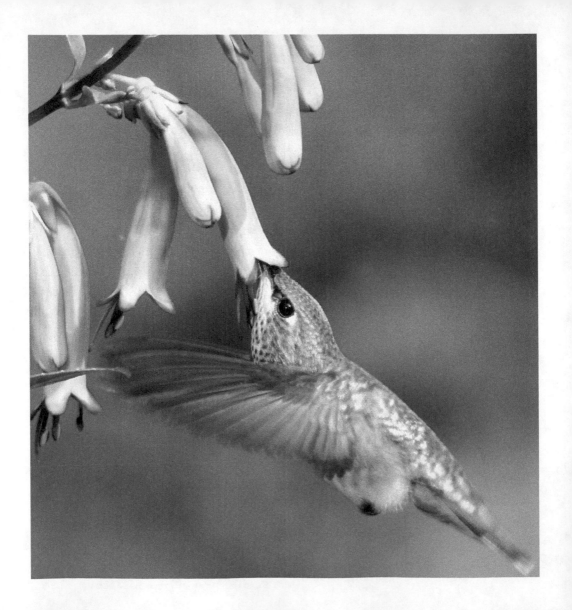

Chancroid is sometimes called a "soft chancre" to distinguish it from the painless chancre of syphilis that feels hard to the touch. If you discover a soft and tender bump, and you have had sexual intercourse during the ten days prior to your detecting this swelling, your partner should be informed immediately, and both of you should be assessed and treated by a medical practitioner.

ECTOPARASITIC INFECTIONS

When your short and curlies turn into a swamp, infested with tiny, itch-causing parasitic bugs such as lice or mites, you are suffering from an ectoparasitic infection. Also known as "crabs," these tiny lice find our curlies a perfectly desirable, warm, and fuzzy home. Fortunately, they are visible to the naked eye and can be treated with a medicinal shampoo, so if you find yourself itching and discover you are hosting tiny lice or nits in your pubic hair, you should advise your partner and seek treatment. You will want to machine wash all of your bedding and clothing in hot water at the same time.

Another ectoparasitic infection, scabies, is caused by a mite that is not visible to the naked eye but can be detected under a magnifying glass or microscope. They crawl all over our skin and cause itching and small bumps and blisters in the webs between the fingers, on the wrists, the back of the elbow, on the knees, in the groin, and on the buttocks. In men, they produce pimplelike bumps on the penis. These tiny, terrorizing creepy-crawlies become especially active at night, which aggravates the itching.

Oral medication can be taken and the body treated with an antiparasitic cream; dramatic itch relief will be experienced after a week or two, but mild itching may persist for up to two months after successful therapy. Furthermore, as with lice, one's sexual partner should also be treated, and all bedding and clothing should be machine washed in hot water.

HUMAN IMMUNODEFICIENCY VIRUS (HIV)
AND ACQUIRED IMMUNODEFICIENCY SYNDROME (AIDS)

The human immunodeficiency virus, or HIV, is a viral infection that weakens the body's immune system and increases the body's vulnerability to many different diseases, including cancer. Primarily, HIV is sexually transmitted but can also be passed on by sharing injection needles used by an infected person, by receiving infected blood, or by infected pregnant women relaying it to their newborn babies. People who have other STDs such as syphilis, genital herpes, chlamydia, gonorrhea, or bacterial vaginosis are at greater risk of contracting HIV. Effective treatment of these diseases reduces the risk of transmission. Condoms are the least expensive and most effective defense in preventing HIV transmission, and male circumcision is said to reduce the risk by 60 percent.

Two to four weeks after becoming infected, nonspecific illnesses such as fever, vomiting, diarrhea, muscle and joint pains, headache, sore throat, or painful lymph nodes may or may not appear. Most people only will test positive twelve weeks after contamination. The average period from exposure to the development of full-blown symptoms is about ten years. These symptoms include unusual illnesses, cancers, tuberculosis, chronic incurable diarrhea, weight loss, intellectual deterioration, dementia, and death. When the symptoms of HIV become this severe, the disease is referred to as acquired immunodeficiency syndrome, or AIDS.

AIDS is one of the most serious and deadly diseases in human history. Although numerous combinations of antiretroviral drugs and drugs that boost the immune system are available for HIV-infected individuals to help control their infection and delay the progression of the disease, there is no cure, which makes prevention so critical.

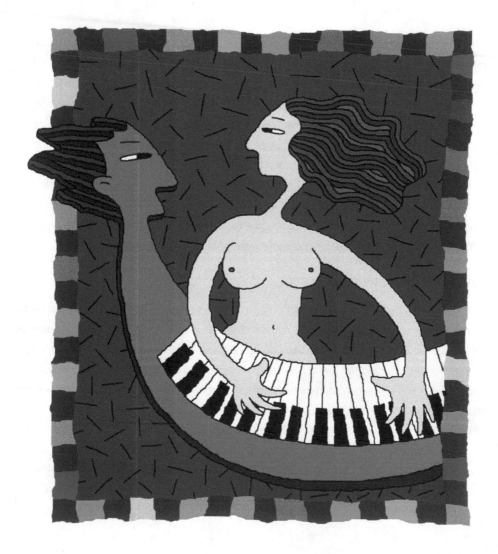

The transmission of HIV from mother to child, however, can be reduced significantly by treating the mother with antiretrovirals during pregnancy and delivery. Sadly only 9 percent of pregnant women with AIDS receive treatment. Infected mothers should refrain from breast-feeding.

The prevalence of HIV/AIDS among women substantially outweighs male incidence: In sub-Saharan Africa, almost 61 percent of adults living with HIV in 2007 were women. To give us any idea of the brutality of this disease, it is imperative to look at more statistics. The number of people living with HIV has risen from 8 million in 1990 to between 33 and 36 million today, and 68 percent of those people live in sub-Saharan Africa. More than 25 million people have died of AIDS since 1981; a rate of almost a thousand fatalities per day, leaving behind at least 11.6 million AIDS orphans in Africa alone. South Africa is home to an estimated 1.4 million of these orphans, and this figure is predicted to rise to 2.5 million by the year 2018.

PELVIC INFLAMMATORY DISEASE (PID)

When the cervix is exposed to a sexually transmitted infection (STI) such as gonorrhea or chlamydia, the bacteria travel up into the internal organs and cause pelvic inflammatory disease (PID). PID is an infection of the female reproductive organs, which include the uterus, Fallopian tubes, and ovaries. These germs, which are transported in the semen and other body fluids of an infected partner, can also contaminate the glands at the opening of the vagina, the urethra (passageway for urine), or the anus.

PID produces different symptoms in different women or, terrifyingly, no symptoms at all. The inauspicious signs of PID do, however, include a dull pain and tenderness in the lower abdomen, lower-back pain, painful urination, a yellow or green vaginal discharge with an unpleasant smell, irregular menstrual periods, painful sex, chills or high fever, nausea, diarrhea, and vomiting.

If you have been exposed to any STDs or suffer from any of these symptoms, consult a doctor without delay. During a pelvic examination, medical personnel will take a swab for analysis and prescribe medication to deter the harmful spread of the infection. Depending on the severity of the infection, you may be treated with antibiotics as an outpatient or be hospitalized. Once the origin of the infection is determined, it is important that your partner also receives treatment to avoid future contamination. Risk factors associated with PID include being sexually active under the age of twenty-five, having multiple sexual partners, and douching habitually.

FINAL COOKIE CRUMBS

Apart from the odd thrush or bacterial vaginosis that many women will experience at some point or another, most sexually transmitted diseases are the result of irresponsible sexual activities. As women, we are known for the gentle hills, fragrant forests, and fertile valleys that our bodies have to offer; to protect that body you must be uncompromising when it comes to sexual discretion.

And that's the way the cookie crumbles....

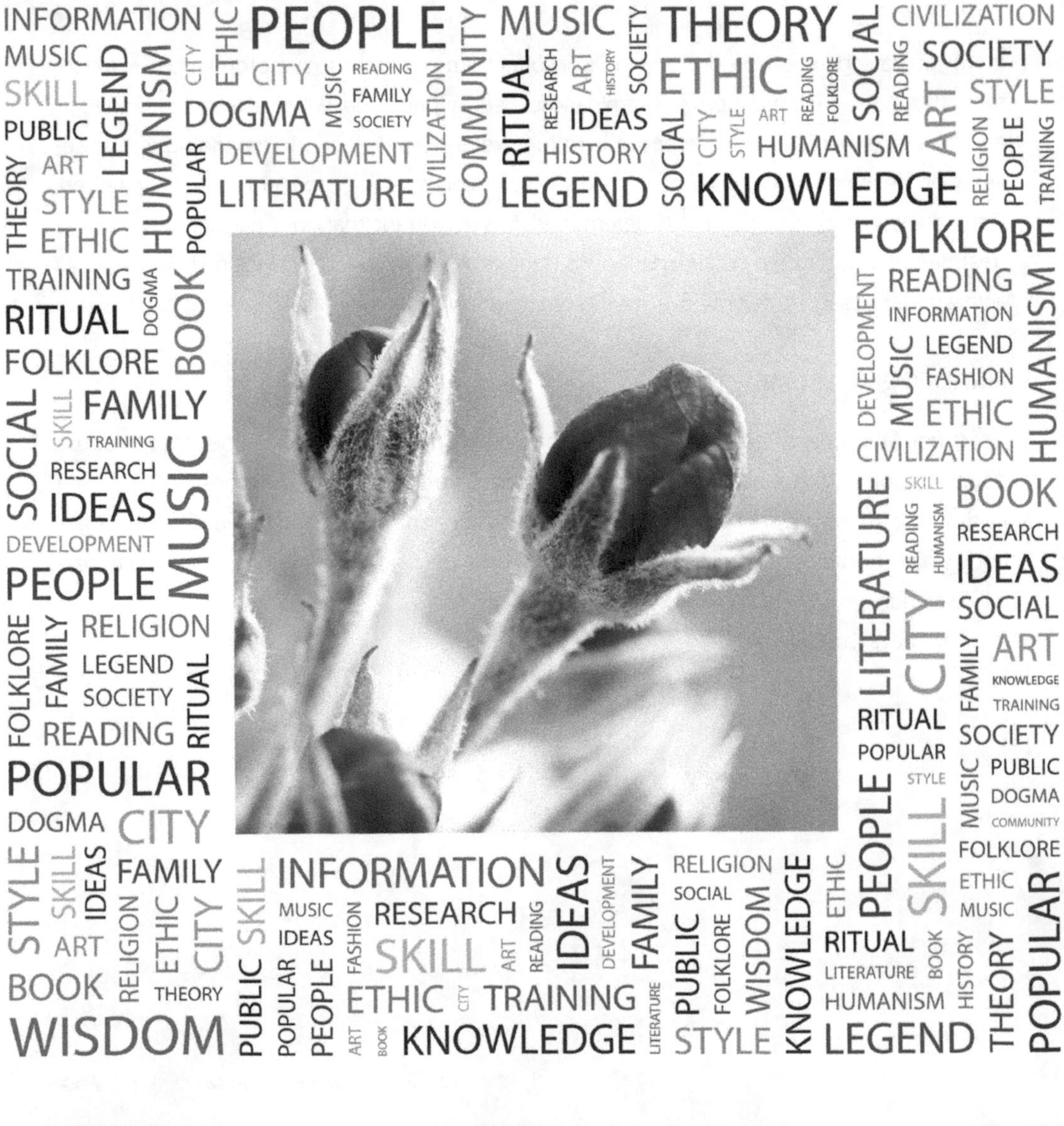
INFORMATION
ETHIC
PEOPLE
COMMUNITY
MUSIC
SOCIETY
THEORY
SOCIAL
CIVILIZATION
MUSIC
CITY
LEGEND
HUMANISM
CITY
READING
FAMILY
SOCIETY
MUSIC
DOGMA
CIVILIZATION
RITUAL
RESEARCH
ART
HISTORY
IDEAS
ETHIC
READING
FOLKLORE
ART
READING
SOCIETY
STYLE
SKILL
PUBLIC
DEVELOPMENT
HISTORY
CITY
STYLE
HUMANISM
ART
RELIGION
PEOPLE
TRAINING
THEORY
ART
STYLE
ETHIC
POPULAR
LITERATURE
LEGEND
SOCIAL
KNOWLEDGE
FOLKLORE
TRAINING
DOGMA
BOOK
READING
RITUAL
DEVELOPMENT
INFORMATION
HUMANISM
FOLKLORE
MUSIC
LEGEND
FASHION
SOCIAL
SKILL
FAMILY
TRAINING
ETHIC
RESEARCH
CIVILIZATION
IDEAS
MUSIC
SKILL
BOOK
DEVELOPMENT
LITERATURE
READING
HUMANISM
RESEARCH
IDEAS
PEOPLE
SOCIAL
CITY
FOLKLORE
FAMILY
RELIGION
FAMILY
ART
LEGEND
KNOWLEDGE
SOCIETY
TRAINING
READING
RITUAL
RITUAL
SOCIETY
POPULAR
POPULAR
PUBLIC
STYLE
DOGMA
DOGMA
CITY
PEOPLE
SKILL
MUSIC
COMMUNITY
FOLKLORE
STYLE
SKILL
IDEAS
FAMILY
INFORMATION
IDEAS
DEVELOPMENT
FAMILY
RELIGION
ETHIC
ART
RELIGION
ETHIC
CITY
SKILL
MUSIC
RESEARCH
READING
SOCIAL
WISDOM
KNOWLEDGE
ETHIC
MUSIC
IDEAS
FASHION
SKILL
ART
PUBLIC
FOLKLORE
RITUAL
BOOK
HISTORY
THEORY
POPULAR
BOOK
THEORY
PUBLIC
POPULAR
PEOPLE
ETHIC
CITY
TRAINING
LITERATURE
LITERATURE
HUMANISM
WISDOM
ART
BOOK
KNOWLEDGE
STYLE
LEGEND

CULTURAL NORMS
AND CUSTOMS

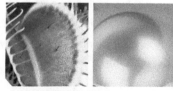
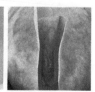

CHAPTER 17

COOKIES WITH A BITE

Dearest Eves and lovers of Eves, in this book we have marveled at our unique anatomy, learned about the life cycle of our vaginas, toyed with hairstyles, and gained valuable information on sexually transmitted diseases. To end our amazing journey, we'll shine a light into the darkest corners of the myths, legends, belief systems, and cultural differences that surround us and reveal how these factors influence and shape our views, behavior, and sexual identity.

The celebrated myth of the *vagina dentata*, or toothed vagina, has been chewing its way into susceptible minds for decades. Throughout the years, this terrifying tale has traveled across the world, striking fear in the hearts of many. In some folk legends, these toothed intimates were rumored to be detached organs, fully capable of crawling around and attacking misbehaving male appendages. In fact, according to a myth of the Mehinaku people of Brazil, *all* women's vaginas previously wandered about. Well, at least until Tukwi, a lady whose vagina would creep around the house looking for porridge and fish stew while she slept, was spotted, caught, and then brutally burned.

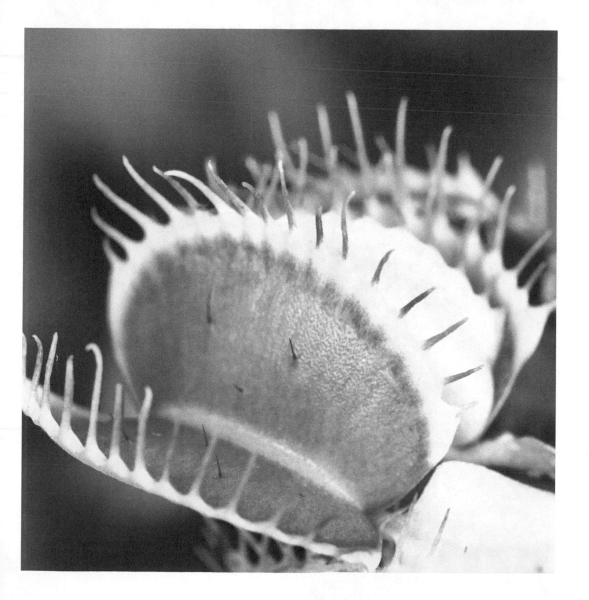

Other folklore warned against hungry dragons or voracious vaginal eels hidden in our intimate crevice. Among the Tembu, a Xhosa-speaking tribe in South Africa, it was believed that women with strong sexual appetites could attract demonic serpents that would come and live in their vaginas, bestowing upon them great pleasure. These snakes could also be sent out to bite men.

In Japan, where the vagina is more gently referred to as the "gate of jewels," it was believed until the nineteenth century that women carried a pearl inside their *ooh-la-las* and that if it were removed, it would cause certain death.

We, as modern-day women living in a contemporary world, don't have the desire to emasculate or mutilate our invited guests. Our vaginas don't harbor dangerous creatures, and we are most certainly not hiding a set of troublesome teeth. In fact, the vagina is a spectacularly sensitive muscular organ, between 3 and 5 inches in length. Rumors of vaginal muscle control have slipped into the history books—Ancient Greece's courtesans, the hetaira, as proof of their genital strength and ability, were famed for being able to crush a clay phallus with their vaginal muscles. This talent for extraordinary vaginal control is also ascribed to Diane de Poitiers, the

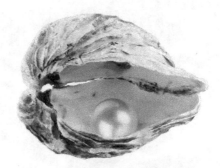

mistress of King Henry II of France (1499–1566), and it is said that Wallis Simpson's "squeeze" was one of the reasons why Britain lost a king in 1936 — it was noted that she had the ability "to make a matchstick feel like a Havana cigar."

BELIEVE IT OR NOT

Ladies, please cross your legs.
All right folks, now that the gates of Hell are closed,
I can begin my sermon.
— Preacher in Idaho, 1920

For centuries, Christian churches believed that sexual intercourse was designed for procreation and procreation alone. Sex was "contrary to natural law" and therefore sinful. In England during the twelfth and thirteenth centuries, the dirty deed was declared illegal on Sundays, Wednesdays, and Fridays, as well as for forty days before both Easter and Christmas.

Outlandish belief systems are not found only in the past. As recently as 1996, British women could take out insurance against fertilization by extraterrestrial beings. Encouraged by the interest shown (more than three hundred women signed up during the first week), the insurance company extended the cover to "virgin conception by an act of God." Even today, some inhabitants of rural Mwanza, Tanzania, claim that HIV/AIDS, like many other illnesses, is caused by bad luck, witchcraft, ancestral spirits, or infected condoms supplied by white people.

We need to recognize that these foreign belief systems, as well as our very own set of values, are derived from our ethnic, historical, socioeconomic, geographic, and political background. Our sexuality, the way we think about our bodies, and our behavior are deeply embedded in the customs that our cultural setting represents.

CHAPTER 18

VARIETY: THE SPICE OF LIFE

The world is filled to the brim with the most incredible characters: the good, the bad, and everything imaginable in between. And because it takes all kinds of people to make the world as diverse as it is, there is an abundance of different practices and beliefs found in history and across cultures—some of which we may view as strange, or even a little bizarre.

For instance, some societies are polygenic (one husband for various wives), some polyandrous (a wife with various husbands), and others monogamous (only one spouse at any given time). In many societies of Melanesia, especially in Papua New Guinea, same-sex relationships formed an integral part of the culture until the middle of the last century. Today same-sex marriages are enjoyed in at least ten countries worldwide, while a number of countries are hostile toward relationships between two people of the same gender. Apart from being illegal in several Muslim nations, same-sex intercourse can, according to the International Lesbian, Gay, Bisexual, Trans and Intersex Association (ILGA), even warrant the death penalty.

We also find the length of foreplay varies between different nations: It may vary from being sharply curtailed or absent to lasting several hours, as in the case of the followers of the

Eastern Tantric tradition. In East Asia, a region known best for Kung Fu and Chinese cuisine, it is reported that one third of Chinese women have never experienced an orgasm, that many make love with their clothes on, and that sexual intercourse often lasts less than a minute. The Australian Aranda and the Chaga from Tanzania are said to engage in sexual intimacy at least three times during one night, while others, like the Keraki women in New Guinea, may abstain from intercourse for years after giving birth.

Kissing on the mouth, which is typically seen as the universal source of sexual arousal, is absent in the Eskimo people of North America and the inhabitants of the Trobriand Islands — they prefer to rub noses. The Tonga tribe of Zimbabwe deems kissing as odious behavior, and as for the Hindu people of India, kissing symbolically contaminates the act of sexual intercourse.

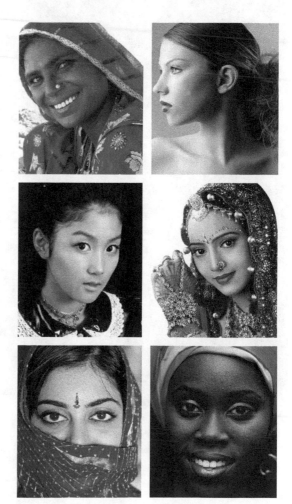

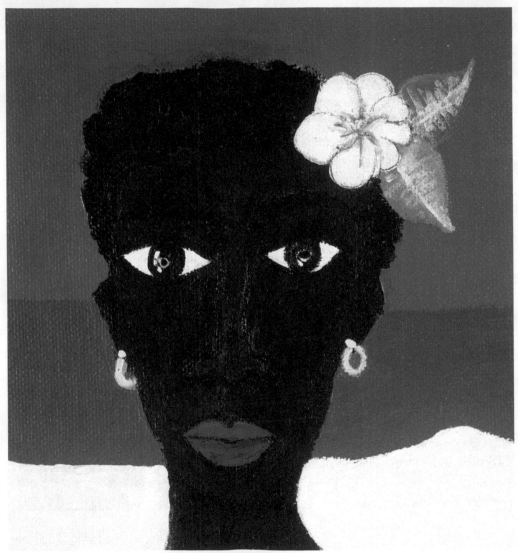

Arnold Rice, *A Flower in Her Hair*

While vaginal lubrication is characteristically seen as a sign of arousal and a prerequisite for sexual intercourse in many places, in some parts of sub-Saharan Africa, like Zambia, Mozambique, and Zimbabwe, it is associated with promiscuity and disease. Because of this belief, a number of practices aim to dry out the vagina prior to sexual intercourse. Substances such as stones, dried leaves, roots, tree bark, baboon urine mixed with soil, alum powders, or rolled-up brown paper are used before sex to dry out the vagina.

In Burkina Faso (West Africa), just a little further north on the map, a more pleasant ritual, in which women eat a porridge-and-root mixture in preparation for marriage, is performed to increase lubrication and to perfume the vagina. Other interesting practices to enhance the "flavor and taste" of the vagina include placing a cotton wool plug drenched in a snuff infusion into the vagina a short while before sexual interaction. This is said to help with the man's erection and to keep him "addictively" faithful.

In some tribal groups in western Kenya, sexual intercourse is used as a sacred rite in a cleansing ritual. According to the Luo's traditional beliefs, a widow becomes unclean subsequent to the death of her husband, so after a year's mourning, an appointed cleaner is hired to sexually cleanse her and restore her place in the community. A feast with friends (and an alcoholic brew) is enjoyed, after which the widow, who would have a woven rope made from banana fibers tied to her waist to denote her unclean status and bond to the deceased, is left alone with the cleanser. The process begins with the two of them shaving each other's pubic hair, followed by sexual relations. If the woven rope breaks, it symbolizes the removal of the sin of death, and the discharge of semen is representative of the cleansing of evil spirits.

CHAPTER 19

FEMALE GENITAL MUTILATION

Another strange but more horrific cultural practice is female genital mutilation (FGM). This term describes the ritualistic practices of cutting and/or removing the female sexual organ. Throughout history, the removal or scarring of intimate parts was performed for various reasons. In England, Isaac Baker Brown published a book in 1866 describing his 70 percent success rate in treating female masturbation, hysteria, and epilepsy with this procedure. Although he was expelled from the Obstetrical Society of London for performing procedures without his patients' consent, the notion of female circumcision gained popularity throughout England. In the United States, during the late Victorian vogue for surgical intervention for nearly all health problems, the Orificial Surgical Society (1890–early 1920s) came into being. They maintained that the orifices below the waist caused most diseases. Many articles and a number of books on the subject of female circumcision were published. In 1912 B. E. Dawson stated, "I do feel an irresistible impulse to cry out against the shameful neglect of the clitoris and its hood, because of the vast amount and sickness and suffering which could be saved the gentler sex." Some of the sicknesses that were said to be cured by female circumcision were headaches, "hip joint disease," and hydrocephaly, which is, as we know today, an abnormal buildup of cerebrospinal fluid in the brain, mostly caused by a birth defect, a brain hemorrhage, or a tumor.

Anthropologists record that among the tribes of the upper Amazon River, clitoral excision was carried out in order to fizzle out the burning sexual passion of Amazonian women and to give their husbands a much-needed rest. Slaves in ancient Rome had rings put through their outer labia to ensure that sexual intercourse could not occur. They could, after all, "not be allowed to fall pregnant lest [their] sale price be lowered." In other cultures, FGM is seen as the "mark of adulthood," promoting the prospect for marriage, health, cleanliness, religion, and fertility. The Dogon people of Mali offer another defense for FGM: They believe that babies are born with two souls—one male and one female. A boy's foreskin represents the female soul, and a girl's clitoral hood, the male soul. In an attempt to assume only one physical identity, both boys and girls are circumcised. Today, FGM is performed mostly in Northeastern Africa, the Middle East, North and South America, Indonesia, and Malaysia. According to Amnesty International, which endeavors to protect human rights worldwide, an estimated thirteen million women, at

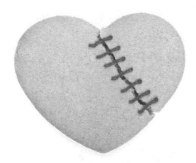

a rate of two million procedures a year, are affected by FGM. This abuse, a travesty of human dignity as the Western world sees it, is often instrumental in attempts to subjugate and manipulate women, and gain control over their sexuality and reproductive health.

FGM is categorized into four general types: clitoridectomy (type I procedure), excision (type II), infibulation (type III), and a type IV procedure that is unclassified but includes all other harmful procedures to the female genitalia. A clitoridectomy is an amputation of the clitoris, or at least parts of it; excision is an amputation of the clitoris and the inner lips of the vagina, and infibulation includes further cuts made to the outer lips of the vagina to produce raw surfaces. These areas are either sewn or clipped together, or joined by tying the legs together to cause the two flaps to fuse and form a "hood" over the vaginal opening. Usually a girl child will be bandaged from hip to ankle so that she remains immobile for approximately forty days to allow for the wound to heal. Only a small opening is left for urination and menstrual discharge. The "hood" of thick skin, or scar tissue, is usually impenetrable and in order to allow for intercourse, our young fellow Eves have to endure manual dilation that causes the skin to tear. Alternatively, the opening may simply be cut open to allow for penetration and childbirth, only to be sewn together again.

Often with no choice or say in the matter, girls between the ages of four and twelve fall victim to this traditional practice. No anesthetic is used, and unsterilized cutting implements such as pieces of glass, blunt pocket knives, or even long nails are often used in unhygienic circumstances. Hemorrhage, septicemia, infertility, and even death are just a few of the physical complications in store for these girls. On a psychological level, many women who survive genital mutilation have an unsurprisingly depressed self-image, lack of confidence, feelings of sexual inadequacy and worthlessness, repressed rage, and anorgasmia (the inability to achieve an orgasm during sexual intercourse).

Although it is difficult to fathom this practice, let alone stand neutral to it, it has to be said that there is something ethically wrong in presenting women of other cultures as victimized, submissive, or ignorant. In some cases, women hold the FGM custom in high esteem and attempts to put a stop to it have foundered because of the fierce tenacity of mothers, grandmothers, and midwives. In Malaysia, for instance, Muslim women in Kelantan feel that it's an important religious requirement, and based on their clinical evidence, women who were subjected to this practice showed no evidence of injury, cutting, scarring, or any form of mutilation to the clitoris. During the procedure, infants are held on their grandmother's lap and only a tiny cut with a razor blade or knife is made to the clitoris. In this case, the term "mutilation" can perhaps be viewed as a misnomer, and it could possibly be considered a symbolic ritual of circumcision rather than mutilation.

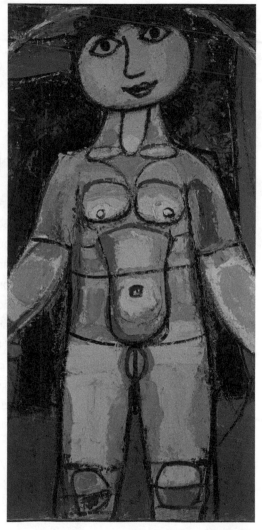

Jean Dubuffet, *A Le Corbusier*

CHAPTER 20

VULVA WORSHIP AND ADORATION

Fascination with the clitoris is by no means new. Our delightful dot is immortalized in stone carvings in the Polynesia's Easter Island in the South Pacific. Here the clitoris demanded special attention and was deliberately lengthened from an early age. During the *te manu mo ta poki* or the "bird child" ceremony, which was still part of living memory in 1919, girls would straddle engraved stones at the ceremonial site of Orongo, displaying their enlarged clitorises to four priests. The girl with the longest clitoris was honored by being carved in stone, and she was granted first option to pick a suitable young man as a partner.

In Hawaii, similar genitalia worship was celebrated in song and dance. Chanting in praise of the genitals, which was part of a song tradition called *mele mai,* was performed in honor of royal babies, and it described and celebrated the vagina's beauty and future capacity. Infants' genitalia were also massaged, stretched, and lengthened in preparation for sexual enjoyment later in life. This positive attitude is reflected in the large lexicon of words for sexual delight and gratification in the Hawaiian language.

Saartjie Baartman, the famous "Hottentot Venus," is a good example of the Khoi Khoi and Khoisan tribes of Southern Africa who believed that large inner labia were a sign of beauty and power. From an early age, the labia would be gently tugged, pulled, and twisted around little sticks and twigs to produce an elongated shape. In 1815, upon Saartjie's death, the renowned French anatomist, Georges Cuvier, described her 4-inch-long inner labia as "two wrinkled, fleshy petals" which, when held apart, created "the figure of a heart." Saartjie's preserved labia were on display in a bell jar in Paris's Musée de l'Homme until the mid 1970s. In 2002, however, on request from President Nelson Mandela, her remains were repatriated to her homeland, the Gamtoos Valley in South Africa.

Elongation of the labia minora is still part of female sexuality practices in the Tete Province of Mozambique and rural northeast Rwanda. This custom is said to highlight feminine beauty; it teaches girls about their own sexuality and prepares them for future sexual relations. The Trukese women of the Carolina Islands displayed a similar positive attitude — fine dangling jewelry and intricate bells were traditionally used as labial piercings.

As part of an agricultural tradition in Japan that dates back more than 1,500 years and is still celebrated today, we find the *Hime-no-Miya Grand Vagina Festival*. During this springtime occasion, children are dressed up beautifully and carry small symbolic vaginas to the Ogata shrine. At the end of a day, filled with prayer and celebration, pink and white *mochi* (glutinous rice ball treats) are hurled into the crowd.

Throughout the years and even today, our vaginas have enjoyed strong cultural interest. In some societies, it is elevated to an almost sacred status, while in others it is downplayed, discarded, or even disgraced. When we as individuals fully ignore or discount these societal beliefs, we risk becoming outcast from our group. While it is not always possible to fully understand various cultural beliefs with their related values and rituals, one must allow for, and respect, the social context in which they exist. This, however, is not to say that harmful cultural norms can't or shouldn't be changed.

TO LOVE AND LEARN

Since the scope of societal diversity is so immense, it is almost impossible to judge what is considered "normal" or what lies outside conventional parameters of belief and behavior. One thing, however, is certain: When we are burdened by negative societal views, we have the opportunity and responsibility to actively change these norms. *We* are the gatekeepers and the caretakers of our intimate treasure.

To understand our quintessential femininity fully and to enjoy self-preservation and empowerment, we need information and open communication. We have to cultivate a love for learning and knowledge, so we need to read, reason, and take some time to discover our own vagina's unique voice. Does she feel neglected and ignored, or recognized and respected? Is she traumatized or safe? Abused or adored? If need be, be courageous and implement gentle changes into your private world: Start conversations with your significant others and be sure to pass on the message of celebration and wonder to your daughters as they undergo this splendid voyage into womanhood.

Protect your most treasured asset from harm and pamper it with love and care. Be proud; there is no need for shameful whispers. The vagina is a miraculous gift, and it is inherently delightful and sexy — let it be lived, heard, and celebrated!

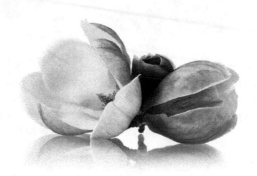

Desert Woman
Janice Cameron

O, desert woman
you patiently wait
to lose weight
to tongue that mouth
to smoke dope
to find that story
to eat cake
to look in the mirror
to taste first snow
to board that plane
to cry your water

O, desert woman
don't wait
eat your thorns
drink your wine
chant your song
shake your rattle
paint your nails
comb your hair
harvest your garden
straddle your buckskin
bleed your water

O, desert woman
you broke the sleep of the seed!
the surge of sun
melts you
down between your
legs the moisture
drips stars
to the flood of sky
the wildflowers are wet
in your mouth
O, desert woman

GLOSSARY

adolescent years: the transitional stage of physical and mental development that occurs between childhood and adulthood. It involves biological, social, and psychological changes.

AIDS (acquired immunodeficiency syndrome): a viral infection that attacks the immune system of the body and causes disease that destroys the body's ability to fight infections and certain cancers.

alkaline powder: contains a combination of minerals, plant calcium, and tissue salts that assists the body in neutralizing high acid levels that can cause heartburn, aching joints, and food cravings. It has antioxidant and immune-boosting properties.

allele [a-leel]: one of a series of different forms of a specific gene. It is an abbreviation for the word *allelomorph*, which describes the variant or different forms of a gene that determine hereditary variation. If a gene has two different alleles for a single trait, such as blue and brown eyes, the dominant allele, which in this case is brown, will be expressed, while the recessive allele is masked.

ambergris [am-ber-grease]: an opaque, ash-colored secretion of the sperm whale intestine, usually found floating on the ocean.

androgen receptor (AR) gene: provides instructions for making a protein called an androgen receptor. Androgens are hormones that are important for normal male sexual development before birth and during puberty and regulate hair growth and sex drive in both males and females.

anorgasmia: failure or inability to achieve an orgasm during sexual intercourse.

antibiotics: powerful medicines that fight bacterial infections.

anti-inflammatory drug: a medicine that relieves pain, lowers fever, and combats inflammation.

anus: the opening of the rectum to the outside of the body.

apocrine sweat glands: glands, located at the junction of the dermis and subcutaneous fat, that release secretions into hair follicles in the armpits *(axillae)*, around the nipples *(areolae)*, and in the groin.

arthritis: the most common form of degenerative joint disease, resulting from trauma, injury or infections of the joints, or old age.

assisted vaginal birth: a vacuum extraction or forceps delivery to assist with childbirth, as opposed to a spontaneous vaginal birth, which relies solely on the mother's own efforts.

atrophy: in regard to genitals, this is the thinning of the membranes of the vulva, the vagina, and the cervix, along with considerable shrinking and loss of elasticity of the outer and inner genital areas.

bacterial vaginosis: a very common vaginal infection in women of reproductive age that is caused by a variety of bacteria. This infection often produces a vaginal discharge that is thin and milky with a "fishy" odor.

Bartholin's glands: a pair of glands between the vulva and the vagina that produces lubrication in response to stimulation and acts to aid in sexual intercourse; also called the greater vestibular glands.

benign: a medical term used to describe a harmless and nonprogressive growth.

biopsy: the removal of a small sample of tissue from a living person for laboratory examination and analysis.

birth control: a way for women and men to prevent pregnancy.

bladder: a muscular organ in which urine is stored.

blood test: a procedure in which a sample of blood is taken from a patient and analyzed in a laboratory for evidence of infection or disease.

candida: a species of fungus that normally lives in small numbers in the vagina and is also present in the mouth and digestive tract of both men and women.

cardiovascular: the circulatory system comprising the heart and blood vessels. The system carries nutrients and oxygen to the body's tissues and removes dioxide and other wastes.

castoreum [ca-staw-ree-um]: the yellowish secretion of the castor sac of the beaver; in combination with the animal's urine, this is used to scent mark an individual's territory.

celibate: a person who abstains from sexual relations.

B

C

Cervarix: a vaccine designed to protect against certain types of human papillomaviruses.

cervical inflammation: swelling of the lower end of the uterus.

cervix: the narrow, lower portion of the uterus, which projects into the vagina and has a small opening to allow fluids, such as semen and cervical secretions, to exchange.

chef d'œuvre [shay-dervr]: the most outstanding work of a creative artist or craftsman; a masterpiece.

chlamydia: a bacterium that is primarily sexually transmitted and infects genital organs.

climacteric [cli-mac-te-rick]: a period of decreasing reproductive capacity in men and women, culminating in female menopause or male midlife crisis. Although a man remains fertile in this period, it corresponds to a reduction in sexual activity.

clitorectomy: the removal of the entire clitoris and the external and internal folds of skin, or "lips" that protect the vaginal opening.

clitoris [klitta-ris]: the small visible structure at the front of the vulva that extends into the internal cavities of a woman's genitalia. It is responsible for sexual arousal when stimulated.

cognitive capabilities: the mental processes of perception, memory, judgment, and reasoning, as contrasted with emotional and volitional processes.

coitus [koy-it-us]: the act of sexual intercourse.

collagen [kolla-jen]: the principal protein of the skin, tendons, cartilage, bone, and connective tissue.

conception: the fertilization of an egg (ovum) by a sperm.

condom: a device, usually made of latex or polyurethane, that is used for birth control and to prevent the spread of sexually transmitted diseases. Male condoms are fitted over the erect penis. Female condoms are inserted into the vagina; the closed end of the condom covers the cervix and the open end covers the area around the opening of the vagina.

connective tissue: a group of supporting body tissues that connects fat, muscle, blood vessels, nerves, bones, and cartilage.

contraceptive: a device or medication that serves to prevent conception or impregnation.

D

daya: a person who has divine qualities and a moral virtue highly prized in all religious and traditional practices.

defloration: the act of losing one's virginity.

diabetes: a condition of the body where sugar is not used correctly to provide energy for living and growing. Diabetes develops when the pancreas doesn't produce enough insulin, which the body needs to produce energy from food.

diagnosis: identification of a disease from signs, symptoms, laboratory tests, radiological results, and physical findings.

diaphragm: a round piece of flexible rubber with a rigid rim used by women for birth control. It is placed in the vagina and against the cervix to prevent semen from entering the womb.

douche: a stream of water directed into the vagina for cleansing or medicinal purposes.

dysmenorrhea: the medical term for the painful cramps that may occur during a woman's menstrual period.

embryology (adjective – **embryological**)**:** the scientific study of embryos and their development.

E

endometriosis: disorder in which tissue similar to that lining the uterus is found growing elsewhere in the body, causing pain and infertility.

epilepsy: a neurological condition that is also known as a seizure disorder.

episodic memory: memory of autobiographical events such as times, places, and faces.

estrogen: a hormone present in both men and women. Estrogen is present in women in significantly higher levels since it promotes the development of female secondary sexual characteristics, such as breasts. Estrogen is also involved in the regulation of the menstrual cycle, which controls fertility. It is also known as the female sex hormone.

excision: the complete removal of an organ, tissue, or a tumor from a body.

Fallopian tubes: two, thin muscular extensions on each side of the uterus connected to the ovaries; the passageway for the female reproductive cell (the ovum, or egg) to travel from the ovaries to the uterus.

F

female circumcision: the removal of part of a female's external genitalia, also known as female genital mutilation.

fertility: the natural capability of giving life; to be able to "to make a baby."

fixatives: in perfumery, it refers to a natural or synthetic substance used to reduce the evaporation rate and improve the stability of a product. Natural fixatives such as sandalwood and musk have a fragrance and are considered base notes in perfumery terms.

frenulum: the underside of the penis, between the shaft and glans.

G

Gardasil: a vaccine approved and recommended by the FDA (U.S. Food and Drug Administration) since September 2009 that protects against certain forms of human papillomaviruses.

genital warts: growths or bumps on the penis, vagina, vulva, cervix, rectum, or groin that are spread by a sexually transmitted virus.

genitalia: the collective term for the anatomical parts of the body that are involved in sexual reproduction.

glans: enlarged, conic structure at the tip of the penis, or the visible tip of the clitoris.

gout: a disease, also known as "the disease of kings," or the "rich man's disease." Elevated levels of uric acid in the bloodstream form crystallized deposits on the cartilage of the joints, the tendons, and the surrounding tissues. It is marked by transient, painful attacks of acute arthritis.

gynecologist: a medical specialist who deals primarily with women's reproductive health.

H

hemorrhage: the loss of blood; bleeding.

HIV test: used to detect the presence of the human immunodeficiency virus in blood, saliva, or urine.

hormones: chemicals released by one or more cells that affect cells in other parts of the body.

hot flashes: sensations of heat that may be accompanied by a red, flushed face and perspiration; the most common complaint of perimenopausal and postmenopausal women.

hysterectomy: the surgical removal of the uterus through either the vagina or an incision in the lower abdomen.

I

ibuprofen: a nonsteroidal, anti-inflammatory drug that relieves symptoms of arthritis, dysmenorrhea, and fever. It is on the World Health Organization's "essential drug list," which specifies the minimum medical needs for a basic health-care system.

immune system: a system of cells that protects the body from bacteria, viruses, toxins, and other foreign substances; this system is the body's natural defense against infection or disease.

induced menopause: immediate menopause caused by medical intervention that removes or damages the ovaries.

infancy: the term derives from the Latin word, *infans*, which means "unable to speak." It is typically applied to children between the ages of one month and twelve months, but it may also include the time between birth and three years of age.

infections: the detrimental colonization of a foreign species, like a parasite, fungi, and viruses, in a host organism. The host organism's response to an infection is inflammation.

infertility: the biological inability of a person to contribute to conception. It also refers to the state of a woman who is unable to carry a pregnancy to full term.

insomnia: a symptom of any of several sleeping disorders. It is characterized by an inability to fall asleep or the persistent inability to sleep for long periods. It affects both the quality and the quantity of sleep.

K-Y Jelly: a water-based, water-soluble personal lubricant; widely used as a sexual aid.

K

L

labia majora: two large, fleshy folds of skin that extend downward from the upper tip of the vulva to the perineum. Each labium has two surfaces: an outer, which is pigmented and covered with hair, and an inner smooth surface leading to the labia minora.

labia minora: small frilly "lips," or folds, that lie inside the labia majora and surround the openings to the urethra and vagina.

laparoscopy: a procedure in which the doctor inserts a small device through an incision in the abdomen in order to view the reproductive organs and pelvic cavity. A sample of tissue may also be collected for testing.

liver spots: also known as "sun spots." These blemishes on the skin are associated with sun exposure and aging. They range in color from light brown to red or black and are located in areas most often exposed to the sun, particularly the hands, face, shoulders, arms, forehead, and the top of the head, if bald.

manganese: an essential trace nutrient present in all forms of life and used in some enzyme reactions for the proper development of bones and cartilage.

M

menopause: signals the end of the fertile phase of a woman's life when menstruation diminishes and ceases; absence of menstrual periods for twelve consecutive months.

menorrhagia: heavy menstrual bleeding.

menstruation: the monthly process whereby the uterine lining is shed, discarding blood and other matter from the womb. Menstruation occurs between puberty and menopause in women who are not pregnant.

mite: a tiny, eight-legged creature, belonging to the order Acarina, that is related to spiders and ticks. Some are parasitic, carry disease, and cause allergies and infection in humans.

mucosa: the moist tissue that lines some organs and cavities throughout the body, including the nose, mouth, lungs, reproductive organs, and digestive tract.

mucous membrane: the lining of various body cavities that is involved in absorption and secretion. The sticky, thick fluid secreted by the mucous membrane is usually called mucus.

N

naproxen: a nonsteroidal, anti-inflammatory drug used to reduce moderate to severe pain, fever, and inflammation.

night sweats: hot flashes that occur during the night.

O

osteoporosis: a condition in which a person loses bone mass and density, causing bones to become fragile or "thin."

ovum (plural: **ova**)**:** female reproductive cell, or egg.

P

pandemic: an epidemic of infectious disease that spreads through human populations across a large region, e.g., a continent or even worldwide.

patriarchal societies: a structure of family units based on the primary authority of the man over the rest of the family members. This authority often includes acting as the dominant figure in social, economic, and political procedures, including serving as the representative via public office.

pelvic cavity: the space inside the pelvis that holds the reproductive organs.

pelvic examination: an examination during which a doctor inserts a speculum (an instrument that widens the vagina) to inspect the vagina, cervix, and uterus for any lumps or changes.

penetration: the insertion of an erect penis into a woman's vagina.

penicillin: an antibiotic derived from *Penicillium* fungi; effective in the treatment of bacterial infections such as syphilis.

perimenopause: the four to six years immediately prior to natural menopause, i.e., not caused by any medical intervention, when changes begin to take place in a women's body in preparation for menopause.

perineum: the tissue between the opening of the rectum and the external genitalia.

pH: an international scale to measure the acidity or basicity of a solution.

pheromones: chemical signals that trigger a natural response in another member of the same species.

physician: a medical specialist who diagnoses and treats diseases and injuries using methods other than surgery.

pneumonia: an infection of one or both lungs that is usually caused by bacteria, viruses, or fungi. Prior to the discovery of antibiotics, 30 percent of people who developed pneumonia died from the infection.

postmenopausal: the years following menopause.

premature menopause: the natural occurrence of menopause before age forty.

progesterone: a female hormone that prepares the uterus to receive a fertilized egg.

prognosis: chance of recovery from an injury or disease.

pubic lice: tiny, six-legged parasitic insects, also called crabs, that typically spread through sexual contact. Humans and gorillas are the only known hosts of this parasite.

quinolone: a synthetic, broad-spectrum antibiotic used in the treatment of gonorrhea.

Q

risk factor: a factor that increases a person's chance of developing a disease, or predisposes a person to a certain condition.

R

semen: the fluid ejaculated through the end of the penis when a man reaches sexual climax.

septicemia: refers to the presence of organisms that cause disease; it often leads to sepsis, a serious medical condition that inflames the whole body.

S

sexual dysfunction: the failure during any phase of the sexual response cycle that prevents the individual or couple from experiencing satisfaction through sexual activity.

sexual health: the many factors that impact sexual function and reproduction. These include a variety of physical, mental, and emotional issues. Disorders that affect any of these factors can influence a person's physical and emotional health, relationships, and self-image.

sexual response cycle: the sequence of physical and emotional changes that occurs as a person becomes sexually aroused and participates in sexually stimulating activities, including intercourse and masturbation.

sexually transmitted disease (STD): a disease passed from one person to another by unprotected sexual contact and activity that involve the mouth, the anus, the penis, and the vagina.

spermicides: foams, jellies, tablets, or suppositories placed in the vagina and up next to the cervix (the opening leading from the vagina to the womb) before sexual intercourse to prevent pregnancy. Spermicides block the cervix and paralyze the sperm, making them unable to travel into the womb.

spotting: light bleeding between menstrual periods.

surgical menopause: instant menopause occurring at any age as a result of surgical removal of the ovaries. Whether menopause is surgical or natural, it can cause symptoms such as hot flashes and night sweats. Sometimes called "sudden menopause."

systemic: means "affecting the entire body" rather than a single organ or body part. Systemic disorders such as high blood pressure, or an infection that is in the bloodstream, are called a systemic infection.

T

tampons: a cylindrical plug of cotton or rayon, or a mixture of the two, inserted into the vagina during menstruation to absorb blood.

testosterone: the male hormone essential for sperm production and the development of male characteristics, including muscle mass and strength, fat distribution, bone mass, facial hair growth, voice change, and sex drive.

toxic shock syndrome (TSS): an acute, potentially fatal circulatory failure, commonly associated with high absorbency tampons that may cause the growth of a toxin-producing bacterium.

trichomonad: a microscopic parasite that can live in the vagina.

ulcer: the appearance of an open sore in the mucous membranes of the body such as on the lips and in and around the genitals.

urethra: the tube that carries urine from the bladder to outside of the body.

urinary tract infection (UTI): occurs when bacteria from outside the body enter the urinary tract and cause infection and inflammation.

uterine contractions: the tightening and shortening of the uterine muscles that occur during labor, the menstrual cycle or in the presence of an infection of the uterine tract.

uterine prolapse: weakening of the tissues that normally hold the uterus in place in the pelvis, allowing it to slip into the vagina.

uterus: also called the womb; a hollow, muscular, pear-shaped organ located in a woman's lower abdomen where fetuses grow and develop.

vaginal atrophy: thinning of the lining of the vagina due to a decline in estrogen that causes dryness, itching, and painful intercourse.

vaginal lubrication: the fluids produced during the sexual arousal phase that reduce friction during sexual intercourse.

vaginitis: a medical term used to describe various disorders that cause infection or inflammation of the vagina.

virus: a microorganism — a germ — which causes various infections.

vulva: all the externally visible parts of female genitalia, including the mons veneris, labia majora, labia minora, clitoris, urethral orifice, and the vaginal vestibule (opening).

yeast infections: infections of the vagina caused by one of the many species of fungus called *Candida*. A change in the chemical balance in the vagina allows the fungus to grow too rapidly, which causes symptoms such as burning and itching.

WORKS CITED

Introduction

P. 1   C. Blackledge, "Vaginas, Les Cons, Weath-er-makers, and Palaces of Delight: Experts from the Story of the V: A Natural History of Female Sexuality," in *Everything You Know about Sex Is Wrong—the Disinformation Guide to the Extremes of Human Sexuality, and Everything in Between*, ed. R. Kick (New York: The Disinformation Company, 2006), 268.

Chapter 1: Naming Our Soft Spot

P. 4   J. Drenth, *The Origin of the World: Science and Fiction of the Vagina*. Translated by Arnold and Erica Pomerans (London: Reaction Books, 2005), 10.

P. 4   C. Jayne, "The Dark Continent Revisited: An Examination of the Freudian View of Female Orgasm," *Psychoanalysis and Contemporary Thought* 3 (1980): 545.

P. 5   S. Pinker, *The Stuff of Thought: Language as a Window into Human Nature* (New York: Penguin Group, 2007), 350.

P. 5   V. Braun and C. Kitzinger, "Snatch, Hole, or Honey-Pot? Semantic Categories and the Problem of Nonspecificity in Female Genital Slang," *Journal of Sex Research* 38, no. 2 (2001): 146–158.

P. 7   "Google Translate," http://translate.google.com/?hl=af# (accessed September 2009); D. Driggs and K. Risch, "Hot Pink: The Girls' Guide to Primping, Passion, and Pubic Fashion," http://ebooks.ebookmall.com/ebook/117270-ebook.htm (accessed 14 November 2009), 56–57; En.Organisasi.Org Community and Library Online, "Vagina in Other Language than English—Online Translation Dictionary," http://en.organisasi.org/translation/vagina-in-other-languages (accessed 19 June 2011); *Collins English-Polish Dictionary*, http://www.credoreference.com.ez.sun.ac.za/book/collinsengpol (accessed 21 June 2011); *Collins German Dictionary*, http://www.credoreference.com.ez.sun.ac.za/vol/529 (accessed 19 June 2011); *Collins French Dictionary Plus*, http://www.credoreference.com.ez.sun.ac.za/vol/503 (accessed 19 June 2011); *Collins Italian Dictionary*, http://www.credoreference.com.ez.sun.ac.za/vol/511 (accessed 21 June 2011);

J. Whitlam, *Collins Dictionary: English-Por-tuguese, Portugues-Ingles*, http://www.credoreference.com.ez.sun.ac.za/vol/501 (accessed 19 June 2011); J. Butterfield, *Collins Spanish Dictionary*, http://www.credoreference.com.ez.sun.ac.za/vol/514 (accessed 21 June 2001); F. Kogos, *A Dictionary of Yiddish Slang and Idioms* (New York: Citadel Press, 1995), 161.

Chapter 2: By the Looks of Things

P. 9   S. Williamson and R. Nowak, "The Truth about Women," New Scientist 159, no. 2145 (1998): 34–35.

P. 10   S. Kitzinger, *Woman's Experience of Sex* (Johannesburg: Flower Press, 1985), 42–43.

P. 13   D. Delvin and C. Webber, "The G-Spot," http://www.netdoctor.co.uk/healthyliving/gspot.htm (accessed 19 August 2008), 13–21.

P. 14   A. V. Burri, L. Cherkas, and T. D. Spector, "Genetic and Environmental Influences on Self-Reported G-Spots in Women: A Twin Study," *Journal of Sexual Medicine* 7, no. 5 (2010): 1842–52.

P. 14   T. Cornforth, "The Clitoral Truth: An Interview with Author Rebecca Chalker," July 17, 2009, http://womenshealth.about.com/cs/sexuality/a/clitoraltruthin.htm (accessed 21 June 2011).

P. 14   D. Sundahl, "Female Ejaculation & the G-Spot," (Alameda, CA: Hunter House, 2003), xvii.

P. 14   C. A. Darling, J. K. Davidson (Sr.), and C. Conway-Welch, "Female Ejaculation: Perceived Origins, the Gräfenberg Spot/Area, and Sexual Responsiveness," *Archives of Sexual Behavior* 19, no. 1 (1990): 29–47.

P. 14   G. L. Gravina, F. Brandetti, P. Martini, E. Carosa, S. M. Di Stasi, S. Morano, A. Lenzi, and E. A. Jannini, "Measurement of the Thickness of the Urethrovaginal Space in Women with or without Vaginal Orgasm," *Journal of Sexual Medicine* 5, no. 3 (2008): 610–18.

P. 14   S. M. A. Thabet, "Reality of the G-Spot and Its Relation to Female Circumcision and Vaginal Surgery," *Journal of Obstetrics and Gynaecology Research* 35, no. 5 (2009): 967–73.

P. 15   P. Hall, "Sexual Health—Enjoying Sex," http://www.bbc.co.uk/relationships/sex_and_sexual_health/enjsex_gspot.shtml (accessed 18 July 2009).

P. 15   F. Addiego, E. G. Belzer (Jr.), J. Comolli, W., Moger, J. D. Perry, and B. Whipple, "Female Ejaculation: A Case Study," *The Journal of Sex Research* 17, no. 1 (1981): 13–21.

P. 16   P. J. Skoll, "Vaginal Labiaplasty," http://www.plasticsurgeon.co.za (accessed 11 February

2008); S. Braun, "Labial Trim." http://www
.drbraun.co.za/plastic-surgery-procedures
/labial-trim.htm (accessed January 27,
2009).

Chapter 3: Scent of a Woman

P. 19   H. Betts, "Let Us Spray," *The Guardian*, December 6, 2008, www.guardian.co.uk (accessed 26 April 2009).

P. 19   D. McCormack, "All in a Stink about Perfume," http://www2.canada.com (accessed 15 April 2009).

P. 21   Betts, "Let Us Spray."

P. 21   McCormack, "All in a Stink about Perfume."

P. 21   Betts, "Let Us Spray."

P. 22   K. Stern and M. K. McClintock, "Regulation of Ovulation by Human Pheromones," *Nature* 392 (1998): 177–79.

P. 24   H. H. Rubin, *Eugenics and Sex Harmony* (New York: Pioneer Publications, 1938), 190.

P. 25   S. Kuukasjärvi, C. J. P. Eriksson, E. Koskela, T. Mappes, K. Nissinen, and K.J. Rantala, "Attractiveness of Women's Body Odors over the Menstrual Cycle: The Role of Oral Contraceptives and Receiver Sex," *Behavioural Ecology* 15, no. 4 (2004): 579–84.

P. 25   J. V. Kohl and R. T. Francoeur, *The Scent of Eros: Mysteries of Odor in Human Sexuality* (Lincoln: iUniverse, 2002), 86.

Chapter 4: Snatch 22: Honey Pot or Hindrance?

P. 30   E. Ensler, "The Vagina Monologues: The V-Day Edition" (New York: Villard Books, 2008). http://www.scribd.com/doc/30286086/ Eve-Ensler-The-Vagina-Monologues (accessed 27 November 2009), 6.

Chapter 5: Kitty Corner

P. 34   I. Opie and P. Opie, *The Oxford Dictionary of Nursery Rhymes*, 2nd ed. (Oxford: Oxford University Press, 1997), 117.

P. 34   I. Larsson, "Sexual Abuse of Children: Child Sexuality and Sexual Behaviour" trans. Lambert and Tudball, http://www.childcentre .info/research/abusedchil/acf6d9.pdf (accessed 7 May 2009), 10.

P. 36   A. Yates, *Sex without Shame: Encouraging the Child's Healthy Sexual Development* (New York: William Morrow, 2009), http:// www.ipce.info/booksreborn/yates/sex /SexWithoutShame.pdf (accessed 1 May 2009), 12.

P. 36   Larsson, "Sexual Abuse of Children," 9.

P. 37   B. N. Gordon and C. S. Schroeder, *Sexuality: A Developmental Approach to Problems* (New York: Plenum Press, 1995), 5–6.

P. 37   T. Melby, "Childhood Sexuality," *Contemporary Sexuality* 35, no. 12 (2001): 3.

P. 39   Larsson, "Sexual Abuse of Children," 15.

P. 39   Ibid., 6.

P. 40 J. H. Kellogg, "Plain Facts for Old and Young: Embracing History and Hygiene of Organic Life," http://www.gutenberg.org/etext/19924 (accessed 15 May 2009), 294.

P. 41 J. H. Kellogg, *Man the Masterpiece* (London: Henry Camp and Co., 1903), 239.

P. 41 Ibid., 240.

P. 43 J. Stengers and A. van Neck, *Masturbation: The History of a Great Terror*, trans. K. Hoffmann (New York: Palgrave, 2001), 133.

Chapter 6: From Tot to Teen

P. 48 M. K. Surbey, "Family Composition, Stress, and the Timing of Human Menarche," in *Socioendocrinology of Primate Reproduction*, ed. T. E. Ziegler and F. B. Bercovitch, 11–32 (Hoboken, NJ: John Wiley & Sons), http://www.jcu.edu.au/sass/idc/groups/public/documents/staff_profiles/jcuprd_021459.pdf (accessed 28 May 2009).

P. 48 R. Quinlan, "Father Absence, Parental Care and Female Reproductive Development," *Evolution and Human Behavior* 24, no. 6 (2003): 376–90.

P. 49 D. E. Comings, D. Muhleman, J. P. Johnson, and J. P. MacMurray, "Parent–Daughter Transmission of the Androgen Receptor Gene as an Explanation of the Effect of Father Absence on Age of Menarche," *Child Development* 73 (2002): 1046–51.

P. 49 J. Mendle et al., "Family Structure and Age at Menarche: A Children-of-Twins Approach," *Developmental Psychology* 42, no. 3 (2006): 533–42.

P. 49 J. M. Lee et al., "Weight Status in Young Girls and the Onset of Puberty," *Pediatrics* 119, no. 3 (2007): 593.

P. 49 D. Costos, R. Ackerman, and L. Paradis, "Recollections of Menarche: Communication Between Mothers and Daughters Regarding Menstruation," *Sex Roles* 46, no. 1–2 (2002): 49–59.

P. 50 Ibid., 50.

P. 52 "Menarche," http://www.absoluteastronomy.com/topics/Menarche (accessed 18 August 2009).

P. 52 D. Morgan-Mar, "Australian Aboriginal Magic," http://www.sjgames.com/pyramid/sample.html?id=4291 (accessed 9 June 2009).

P. 53 S. Supriya, "Celebrate Womanhood," http://living.oneindia.in/insync/pulse/2006/celebrate-womanhood.html (accessed 24 May 2009).

Chapter 7: On Virgin Territory

P. 54 S. Kitzinger, *Woman's Experience of Sex* (Johannesburg: Flower Press, 1985), 179.

P. 57 J. Drenth, The Origin of the World: Science and Fiction of the Vagina. Translated by

Arnold and Erica Pomerans (London: Reaction Books, 2005), 68.

P. 57   A. J. Hobday, L. Haury, and P. K. Dayton, "Function of the Human Hymen," *Medical Hypotheses* 49, no. 2 (1997): 171–73.

P. 57   S. J. Emans, "Physical Examination of the Child and Adolescent," in *Evaluation of the Sexually Abused Child: A Medical Textbook and Photographic Atlas*, eds. A. H. Heger, S. J. Emans, and D. Muran, 2nd ed. (New York: Oxford University Press, 2000), 64.

P. 58   J. A. Adams, A. S. Botash, and N. Kellogg, "Differences in Hymenal Morphology Between Adolescent Girls with and Without a History of Consensual Sexual Intercourse," *Archives of Pediatrics and Adolescent Medicine* 158, no. 3 (2004): 280.

P. 58   N. D. Kellogg, S. W. Menard, and A. Santos, "Genital Anatomy in Pregnant Adolescents: 'Normal' Does Not Mean 'Nothing Happened,'" *Pediatrics* 113, no. 1 (2004): 67.

P. 59   Drenth, The Origin of the World, 69.

P. 59   Ibid., 69.

P. 59   L. le Roux, "Harmful Traditional Practices: Male Circumcision and Virginity Testing of Girls and the Legal Rights of Children" (Magister Legum thesis, University of the Western Cape, South Africa, 2006), http://etd.uwc.ac.za/usrfiles/modules/etd/docs /etd_gen8Srv25Nme4_8182_1183427422.pdf (accessed 5 February 2009), 13.

P. 60   L. Jamieson and P. Proudlock, "Children's Bill Progress," http://web.uct.ac.za/depts/ci/plr /cbill.htm (accessed 14 May 2009), 15.

P. 60   L. le Roux, "Harmful Traditional Practices," 15.

P. 60   A. Chozick, "US Women Seek a Second First Time with Hymen Surgery," *The Wall Street Journal*, 15 December 2005, http://www .urogyn.org/documents/Hymenoplastyon WSJ.doc (accessed 8 June 2009).

P. 63   R. E. Rector, K. A. Johnson and L. R. Noyes, "Sexually Active Teenagers Are More Likely to Be Depressed and to Attempt Suicide," http://www.heritage.org/Research/Family /cda0304.cfm (accessed 30 May 2009).

Chapter 8: The Effects of Sex on the Vagina

P. 64   "Sexual Response Cycle," http://www. soc.ucsb.edu/sexinfo/article/the-sexual -response-cycle#four (accessed 31 June 2009).

P. 66   "Evolution and Revolution: The Past, Present, and Future of Contraception," *Baylor College of Medicine* 10, no. 6 (2000), http://www.contraceptiononline.org /contrareport/article01.cfm?art=93 (accessed May 29, 2009).

P. 66   Planned Parenthood Federation of

America, *A History of Birth Control Methods* (New York: Katharine Dexter McCormick Library, 2006), http://www.plannedparenthood.org/files/PPFA/history_bc_methods.pdf (accessed 25 June 2011), 6.

P. 68 Ibid., 1.

P. 68 "Evolution and Revolution," http://www.contraceptiononline.org/contrareport/article01.cfm?art=93 (accessed May 29, 2009).

P. 68 H. Youssef, "The History of the Condom," *Journal of the Royal Society of Medicine* 86, no. 4 (1993): 226–28.

P. 69 Ibid., 227.

P. 69 D. J. Brewer and E. Teeter, *Ancient Egyptian Society and Family Life* (Cambridge: Cambridge University Press, 2001), http://www.fathom.com/course/21701778/session2.html (accessed 26 July 2009).

Chapter 9: Pregnancy and Childbirth

P. 70 J. Drenth, *The Origin of the World: Science and Fiction of the Vagina*. Translated by Arnold and Erica Pomerans (London: Reaction Books, 2005), 149.

P. 70 S. Kitzinger, *Woman's Experience of Sex* (Johannesburg: Flower Press, 1985), 203.

P. 71 Ibid., 220.

P. 72 Ibid., 222.

P. 72 V. L. Handa, "Sexual Function and Childbirth," *Seminars in Perinatology* 30, no. 5 (2006): 253–256.

P. 73 C. Phillips and A. Monga, "Childbirth and the Pelvic Floor: The Gynaecological Consequences," *Reviews in Gynaecological Practice* 5, no. 1 (2005): 15–22.

P. 73 Drenth, *The Origin of the World*, 148.

P. 73 Phillips and Monga, "Childbirth and the Pelvic Floor," 15–22.

Chapter 10: A Change of Season

P. 76 G. A. Larue, "Ancient Ethics," in *A Companion to Ethics*, ed. P. Singer (Oxford: Blackwell Publishing, 1993), 30.

P. 79 D. Kingsley, "Early Menopause Is Strongly Genetic," http://www.abc.net.au/science/articles/2001/08/30/354928.htm (accessed 19 July 2009).

P. 79 J. Pascarl, "An Open Letter to Men with Fast Cars and Fancy Watches," http://www.thepunch.com.au/articles/an-open-letter-to-middle-aged-men-with-fast-cars (accessed 15 July 2009).

P. 80 K. L. Giblin, "Sex and Menopause: The Sizzle and the Fizzle," *Sexuality, Reproduction and Menopause* 3, no. 2 (2005): 72–77.

P. 80 C. Castelo-Branco et al., "Management of Post-Menopausal Vaginal Atrophy and Atrophic Vaginitis," *Maturitas* 52, suppl. 1 (2005): 47.

P. 81   M. Freedman et al., "Twice-Weekly Synthetic Conjugated Estrogens Vaginal Cream for the Treatment of Vaginal Atrophy," *The Journal of the North American Menopause Society* 16, no. 4 (2009): 735–41.

P. 81   C. Castelo-Branco et al., "Management of Post-Menopausal Vaginal Atrophy and Atrophic Vaginitis," *Maturitas* 52, suppl. 1 (2005): 46–52.

P. 81   M. S. Walid, "Prevalence of Urinary Incontinence in Female Residents of American Nursing Homes and Association with Neuropsychiatric Disorders," *Journal of Clinical Medicine Research* 1, no. 1 (2009): 37–39.

P. 83   A. L. Olesen et al., "Epidemiology of Surgically Managed Pelvic Organ Prolapse and Urinary Incontinence," *Obstetrics and Gynecology* 89, no. 4 (1997): 501–506.

P. 83   C. M. Meston, "Aging and Sexuality," *Western Journal of Medicine* 167, no. 4 (1997): 285–90.

P. 85   K. O'Hanlan, "Alternative Treatments for Menopausal Symptoms," http://www.ohanlan.com/PDFs/Alternatives_to_estrogen.pdf (accessed 25 July 2009).

P. 85   C. M. Meston, "Aging and Sexuality," *Western Journal of Medicine* 167, no. 4 (1997): 285–90.

P. 85   L. Hansen et al., "Sexual Health," BioMed Central (BMC) Women's Health 4, suppl. 1 (2004): S24.

P. 86   "The Impact of Menopause: Survey Results," http://www.emaxhealth.com/1/70/32545/impact-menopause-survey-results.html (accessed 2 July 2009).

P. 86   "Menopausal Bioidentical Hormones," http://66.246.156.147/for-women/menopausal-bioidentical-hormones (accessed 3 July 2009).

P. 86   "The Impact of Menopause: Survey Results," http://www.emaxhealth.com/1/70/32545/impact-menopause-survey-results.html (accessed 2 July 2009).

P. 86   N. F. Woods, "Exercise, Fitness, and Quality of Life: Implications for Health Promotion for Midlife and Older Women," *The Journal of the North American Menopause Society* 15, no. 4 (2008): 579–80; L. Dennerstein et al., "Modeling Women's Health During the Menopausal Transition: A Longitudinal Analysis," *The Journal of the North American Menopause Society* 14, no. 1 (2006): 53–62; H. Roberts, "Managing the Menopause," *British Medical Journal* 334 (2007): 736–41.

P. 86   D. W. Kaufman et al., "Cigarette Smoking and Age at Natural Menopause," *American Journal of Public Health* 70, no. 4 (1980): 420–22.

P. 86   J. Ginsberg, "What Determines the Age at the Menopause?" *British Medical Journal* 302, no. 6788 (1991): 1288–89.

P. 87   "Andre Maurois Quotes," http://www
.brainyquote.com/quotes/quotes/a
/andremauro158002.html (accessed 22 July
2009).

Chapter 11: Tattooing and Body Piercing

P. 90   J. Levy, *Tattoos in Modern Society* (New York:
Rosen Publishing Group, 2009), 20–22.

P. 90   L. G. Ruscone, "Sailor Tattoos," http://www
.tattoolife.com/archive/arch_16.html (accessed 4 March 2009).

P. 91   J. Kazandjieva, I. Grozdev, and N. Tsankov,
"Temporary Henna Tattoos," *Clinics in Dermatology* 25, no. 4 (2007): 383.

P. 93   "Henna and Mehndi Tattoos: Where It
All Started and Why," http://www.henna
-tattoos-kits.com/henna-tattoo/history
.htm (accessed 14 March 2009).

P. 93   Kazandjieva, Grozdev, and Tsankov, "Temporary Henna Tattoos," 384.

P. 93   W. R. Hesse Jr., *Jewelry Making Through
World History: An Encyclopedia* (London:
Greenwood Press, 2007), xvii and 25.

P. 93   C. Morrison, "Body Piercing History," http://
www.painfulpleasures.com/piercing
_history.htm (accessed 23 February 2008).

P. 93   D. Malloy, "Body and Genital Piercing in
Brief," http://www.bmezine.com/news/jim
ward/20040315-p.html (accessed 13 February 2009).

P. 93   "The History of Jewelry: Ethnic Tribal Jewelry," http://www.khulsey.com/jewelry
/jewelry_history_primitive_ethnic_tribal
.html (accessed 14 January 2009).

P. 93   D. J. Pantone, "The Matis and Matsés Indians of the Amazon Rainforest," http://
www.amazon-indians.org/page02.html
(accessed 27 June 2009).

P. 93   L. M. Koenig, "Body Piercing: Medical Concerns with Cutting-Edge Fashion," *Journal
of General Internal Medicine* 14, no. 6 (1999):
379–85.

P. 94   J. Kazandjieva and N. Tsankov, "Tattoos:
Dermatological Complications," *Clinics in
Dermatology* 25, no. 4 (2007): 376; Koenig,
"Body Piercing: Medical Concerns with
Cutting-Edge Fashion," 379–385.

P. 94   "Tattoo, Piercing and Breast Implantation
Infections," http://www.medicalnewstoday
.com/articles/41238.php (accessed 14 March
2009).

P. 94   Koenig, "Body Piercing: Medical Concerns
with Cutting-Edge Fashion," 379–85.

Chapter 12: Color, Cut, and Curl

P. 96   T. Hamilton, *Skin Flutes and Velvet Gloves:
A Collection of Facts and Fancies, Legends
and Oddities about the Body's Private Parts*
(New York: St. Martin's Press, 2002), 169.

P. 97   H. Hoby, "The Fashion Designer Mary Quant," *The Guardian*, 21 June 2009, http://www.guardian.co.uk/society/2009/jun/21/older-people-fashion-designers (accessed 23 August 2009).

P. 97   "Francisco de Goya Paintings," http://www.paintinghere.com/artist-1/Francisco-de-Goya-Paintings.html (accessed 3 February 2009).

P. 97   J. Batchelor, *John Ruskin: A Life* (New York: Carroll & Graf Publishers, 2000), 127.

P. 97   T. Hilton, *John Ruskin* (Connecticut: Yale University Press, 2002), 117.

P. 99   M. E. Ginway, *Brazilian Science Fiction: Cultural Myths and Nationhood in the Land of the Future* (Cranbury: Associated University Press, 2004), 56.

Chapter 13: Hair Care Down There

P. 105 Uniformed Services University of the Health Sciences, "Deployment Dermatology," http://rad.usuhs.mil/derm/lecture_notes/Norton_deployderm.htm (accessed 13 October 2009).

P. 105 Ibid.

P. 106 D. Driggs and K. Risch, "Hot Pink: The Girls' Guide to Primping, Passion, and Pubic Fashion," http://ebooks.ebookmall.com/ebook/117270-ebook.htm (accessed 14 November 2009), 31.

P. 107 N. Torres, "Ingrown Hair Home Treatment," http://hairremoval.about.com/od/shaving/a/ingrown-home.htm (accessed 25 February 2009).

P. 107 Ibid.

P. 107 N. Torres, "How to Make an Asprin Mask," http://hairremoval.about.com/od/shaving/a/asprin-mask.htm (assessed 25 February 2009)

P. 108 "Anal Bleaching," http://bestanalbleaching.com (accessed 14 March 2009).

Chapter 14: The Wandering Uterus

P. 112 G. R. Smith Jr., *Somatization Disorder in the Medical Setting* (Washington, DC: American Psychiatric Press, 1991), 5.

P. 112 Ibid., 9.

P. 112 Ibid., 10.

P. 112 J. Drenth, The Origin of the World: Science and Fiction of the Vagina, trans. Arnold and Erica Pomerans (London: Reaction Books, 2005), 216.

P. 114 Smith Jr., *Somatization Disorder in the Medical Setting*, 5; M. R. Lefkowitz and M. B. Fant (eds.), *Women's Life in Greece and Rome: A Source Book in Translation*, 2nd ed. (Baltimore, Maryland: Johns Hopkins University Press, 1992), 246.

P. 114 Lefkowitz and Fant, eds., *Women's Life in Greece and Rome*, 246–48.

P. 114   Drenth, The Origin of the World: Science and Fiction of the Vagina, 217.

P. 115   R. P. Maines, "Freud and the Steam-Powered Vibrator," in Longing: Psychoanalytic Musings on Desire, ed. J. Petrucelli (London: H Karnac Books, 2006), 121–25.

P. 115   Smith Jr., Somatization Disorder in the Medical Setting, 7.

Chapter 15: Vaginal Infections

P. 116   M. D. Mazumbar, "Vaginal Discharge without Itching," http://www.gynaeonline.com/vaginitis.htm (accessed 11 August 2009); MedlinePlus, "Vaginal Discharge," http://www.nlm.nih.gov/medlineplus/ency/article/003158.htm (accessed 14 August 2009).

P. 121   P. G. Pappas, "Invasive Candidiasis," Infectious Disease Clinics of North America 20, no. 3 (2006): 485–506; R. Arnsel et al., "Nonspesific Vaginitis: Diagnostic Criteria and Microbial and Epidemiologic Associations," American Journal of Medicine 74, no. 1 (1983): 14–22; MedlinePlus, "Vaginal Yeast Infection," http://www.nlm.nih.gov/medlineplus/ency/article/001511.htm (accessed 14 August 2009); MedlinePlus, "Vaginal Yeast Infection," http://www.nlm.nih.gov/medlineplus/ency/article/001511.htm (accessed 14 August 2009).

P. 121   C. S. Bradshaw et al., "High Recurrence Rates of Bacterial Vaginosis over the Course of 12 Months after Oral Metronidazole Therapy and Factors Associated with Recurrence," Journal of Infectious Diseases 193, no. 11 (2006): 1478–86; R. S. Gibbs, "Asymptomatic Bacterial Vaginosis: Is It Time to Treat?" American Journal of Obstetrics and Gynecology 196, no. 6 (2007): 495–96; Centers for Disease Control and Prevention, "Bacterial Vaginosis: CDC Fact Sheet," http://www.cdc.gov/std/bv/STDFact-Bacterial-Vaginosis.htm#Complications (accessed 2 August 2009).

P. 123   Centers for Disease Control and Prevention, "Trichomoniasis: CDC Fact Sheet," http://www.cdc.gov/std/trichomonas/default.htm (accessed 21 August 2009); S. L. Cudmore et al., "Treatment of Infections Caused by Metronidazole-Resistant Trichomonas Vaginalis," Clinical Microbiology Reviews 17, no. 4 (2004): 783–93.

P. 124   J. Nissl, "Object in the Vagina," http://health.msn.com/health-topics/articlepage.aspx?cp-documentid=100078649 (accessed 27 May 2009); E. C. Nwosu et al., "Foreign Objects of Long Duration in the Adult Vagina," Journal of Obstetrics and Gynaecology 25, no. 7 (2005): 737–39.

P. 124 M. C. Stöppler, "Vaginal Bleeding," http://
www.medicinenet.com/vaginal_bleeding
/article.htm (accessed 27 August 2009);
Q. Newton Long, "Abnormal Vaginal Bleeding," in *Gynecology Principles and Practice*,
ed. R. E. Kirstner, 3rd ed. (Chicago: Book
Medical Publishers, 1979) 810–12; E-Medicine Health, "Vaginal Bleeding," http://www
.emedicinehealth.com/vaginal_bleeding
/article_em.htm (accessed 7 June 2009).

P. 124 "About Endometriosis," http://www.endo
metriosis.org/endometriosis.html (accessed 15 September 2008).

Chapter 16: Sexually Transmitted Diseases

P. 128 Centers for Disease Control and Prevention, "Gonorrhea: CDC Fact Sheet,"
http://www.cdc.gov/std/Gonorrhea
/STDFact-gonorrhea.htm (accessed 27 August 2009); Y. T. H. P. van Duynhoven, "The
Epidemiology of Neisseria Gonorrhoeae
in Europe," *Microbes and Infection* 1, no. 6
(1999): 455–64; M. C. Stöppler, "Gonorrhea
in Women," http://www.medicinenet.com
/gonorrhea_in_women/article.htm (accessed 25 September 2009).

P. 129 Centers for Disease Control and Prevention,
"Chlamydia: CDC Fact Sheet," http://www
.cdc.gov/std/Chlamydia/STDFact-Chlam
ydia.htm (accessed 26 August 2009).

P. 130 Centers for Disease Control and Prevention,
"Syphilis: CDC Fact Sheet," http://www.cdc
.gov/std/syphilis/syphilis-fact-sheet.pdf
(accessed 3 August 2009); M. C. Stöppler,
"Syphilis in Women," http://www.medicine
net.com/syphilis_in_women/page2.htm
(accessed 22 September 2009).

P. 132 Centers for Disease Control and Prevention, "Herpes: CDC Fact Sheet," http://www
.cdc.gov/std/herpes/STDFact-herpes.htm
(accessed 2 August 2009); M. C. Stöppler,
"Genital Herpes in Women," http://www
.medicinenet.com/genital_herpes_in
_women/article.htm (accessed 3 August
2009).

P. 132 J. van Schoor, "Gardasil™: Quadrivalent HPV
Vaccine," *SA Pharmaceutical Journal* 75, no. 4
(2008): 34; Centers for Disease Control and
Prevention, "Human Papillomavirus (HPV)
Infection: CDC Fact Sheet," http://www.cdc
.gov/std/HPV/STDFact-HPV.htm (accessed
3 August 2009); Centers for Disease Control
and Prevention, "Genital Human Papillo
mavirus: CDC Fact Sheet," http://www.cdc
.gov/STD/HPV/STDFact-HPV.htm (accessed
26 August 2009).

P. 133 Medical News Today, "FDA Advisory Committee Makes Favorable Recommendation
for Cervarix, GlaxoSmithKline's Candidate
Cervical Cancer Vaccine," http://www.medi

calnewstoday.com/articles/163453.php (accessed 3 October 2009); MSNBC.com, "FDA Backs New Cervical Cancer Vaccine Cervarix," http://www.msnbc.msn.com/id/32760999/ns/health-sexual_health (accessed 3 October 2009).

P. 133 MedlinePlus, "Chancroid," http://www.nlm.nih.gov/medlineplus/ency/article/000635.htm (accessed 25 October 2009); MERCK, "Chancroid: Sexually Transmitted Diseases," http://www.merck.com/mmpe/sec14/ch194/ch194b.html (accessed 26 October 2009).

P. 135 A. Rockoff and M. C. Stöppler, "Scabies," http://www.medicinenet.com/scabies/article.htm (accessed 27 September 2009); MedicineNet.com, "Pubic Lice (Crabs)," http://www.medicinenet.com/pubic_lice_crabs/article.htm (accessed 4 October 2009); MedicineNet.com, "Scabies: Symptoms, Signs, Treatments and Facts," http://www.medicinenet.com/scabies/page3.htm (accessed 27 September 2009); K. A. Workowski and S. M. Berman, "Ectoparasitic Infections: Sexually Transmitted Diseases Treatment Guidelines," http://www.guideline.gov/summary/summary.aspx?ss=15&doc_id=9687&nbr=5196 (accessed 21 August 2009).

P. 136 L. O. Kallings, "The First Postmodern Pandemic: 25 Years of HIV/AIDS," *Journal of Internal Medicine* 263, no. 3 (2008): 218–43; Joint United Nations Programme on HIV/AIDS, "AIDS Epidemic Update," http://data.unaids.org/pub/EPISlides/2007/2007_epiupdate_en.pdf (accessed 15 September 2009); Joint United Nations Programme on HIV/AIDS, "2008 Report on the Global AIDS Epidemic: Executive Summary," http://data.unaids.org/pub/GlobalReport/2008/JC1511_GR08_ExecutiveSummary_en.pdf (accessed 15 September 2009); AVERT, "Aids Orphans," http://www.avert.org/aids-orphans.htm (accessed 15 September 2009); Centre for Actuarial Research, "The Impact of AIDS on Orphanhood in South Africa: A Quantitative Analysis," http://www.commerce.uct.ac.za/Research_Units/CARE/Monographs/Monographs/mono04.pdf (accessed 23 September 2009); K. A. Sepkowitz, "AIDS: The First 20 Years," *The New England Journal of Medicine* 344, no. 23 (2001): 1764–73; "HIV and AIDS," http://kidshealth.org/teen/sexual_health/stds/std_hiv.html (accessed 5 August 2009).

P. 138 Centers for Disease Control and Prevention, "Pelvic Inflammatory Disease: CDC Fact Sheet," http://www.cdc.gov/std/PID/STDFact-PID.htm (accessed 23 August 2009); "Pelvic Inflammatory Disease," http://www.medicinenet.com/pelvic_inflam

matory_disease/article.htm (accessed 3 October 2009).

Chapter 17: Cookies with a Bite

P. 142 C. Blackledge, *The Story of V: A Natural History of Female Sexuality*. (New Jersey: Rutgers University Press, 2003),165.

P. 142 Ibid., 166

P. 144 Ibid., 168.

P. 144 Ibid., 177.

P. 144 Ibid., 181.

P. 145 Ibid., 182

P. 145 J. Drenth, *The Origin of the World: Science and Fiction of the Vagina*, trans. Arnold and Erica Pomerans (London: Reaction Books, 2005), 255.

P. 145 Blackledge, *The Story of V: a Natural History of Female Sexuality*, 51.

P. 145 Drenth, *The Origin of the World: Science and Fiction of the Vagina*, 103.

P. 145 G. Mshana et al., "She Was Bewitched and Caught an Illness Similar to AIDS: AIDS and Sexually Transmitted Infection Causation Beliefs in Rural Northern Tanzania," *Culture, Health and Sexuality* 8, no. 1 (2006): 45–52.

Chapter 18: Variety: The Spice of Life

P. 146 G. H. Herdt, ed., *Ritualized Homosexuality in Melanesia* (Berkeley, CA: University of California Press, 1993) xv–xviii.

P. 146 ILGA (International Lesbian, Gay, Bisexual, Trans and Intersex Association), "World Day Against Death Penalty," http://ilga.org/ilga/en/article/1111 (accessed 24 August 2011).

P. 147 S. Ubillos, D. Paez, and J. L. González, "Culture and Sexual Behavior," *Psicothema* 12 (2000): 73.

P. 147 R. Crooks and K. Baur, *Sexual Arousal and Response*. 10th ed. (Belmont, California: Thomson Higher Education, 2008), 139.

P. 149 S. Braunstein and J. van de Wijgert, *Cultural Norms and Behavior Regarding Vaginal Lubrication During Sex: Implications for the Acceptability of Vaginal Microbicides for the Prevention of HIV/STIs* (New York: The Population Council, 2003), 6.

P. 149 Ibid., 22.

P. 149 E. Boikanyo, "So Much for Women-Sensitive Sexual Relations: The Use of Vaginal Potions," *Women and Health* 15 (1992): 4.

P. 149 R. Ayikukwei et al., "HIV/AIDS and Cultural Practices in Western Kenya: The Impact of Sexual Cleansing Rituals on Sexual Behaviours," *Culture, Health and Sexuality* 10, no. 6 (2008): 587–99.

Chapter 19: Female Genital Mutilation

P. 150 F. J. Green, "From Clitoridectomies to 'Designer Vaginas': The Medical Construction of Heteronormative Female Bodies and

Sexuality Through Female Genital Cutting,"
Sexualities, Evolution and Gender 7, no. 2
(2005): 162.

P. 150 "Orificial Surgery: The Orificial Surgery
Society and Orthodox Medicine," http://
www.historyofcircumcision.net/index.php
?option=com_content&task=view&id=52
&Itemid=0 (accessed 24 July 2009); Ira M.
Rutkow, "Orificial Surgery" *Archives of Surgery* 136 (Sept. 2001): 1088.

P. 151 C. Blackledge, *The Story of V: A Natural
History of Female Sexuality.* (New Jersey:
Rutgers University Press, 2003), 136.

P. 151 J. Drenth, *The Origin of the World: Science
and Fiction of the Vagina*, trans. Arnold and
Erica Pomerans (London: Reaction Books,
2005), 186.

P. 151 K. E. Paige, "The Ritual of Circumcision,"
Human Nature 1, no. 5 (1978): 40–48.

P. 151 Blackledge, *The Story of V: A Natural History
of Female Sexuality*, 134.

P. 152 A. Lewnes, "Changing a Harmful Social
Convention: Female Genital Mutilation/
Cutting," http://www.unicef-irc.org/publi
cations/pdf/fgm_eng.pdf (accessed 27
February 2009), 1.

P. 152 N. Toubia, "Female Circumcision as a Public
Health Issue," *The New England Journal of
Medicine*, 331, no. 11 (1994): 713–15.

P. 152 H. Lightfoot-Klein, "Prisoners of Ritual:

Some Contemporary Developments in the
History of FGM," http://www.fgmnetwork
.org/Lightfoot-klein/prisonersofritual.htm
(accessed 5 February 2008).

P. 153 Ab. Rahman Isa, R. Shuib, and M. S. Othman, "The Practice of Female Circumcision
Among Muslims in Kelantan, Malaysia,"
Reproductive Health Matters 7, no. 13 (May
1999): 138.

Chapter 20: Vulva Worship and Adoration

P. 154 Blackledge, C. *The Story of V: A Natural
History of Female Sexuality.* (New Jersey:
Rutgers University Press, 2003), 137.

P. 154 Ibid., 139

P. 155 Ibid., 141

P. 155 B. Bagnoli and E. Mariano, "Vaginal Practices: Eroticism and Implications for
Women's Health and Condom Use in Mozambique," *Culture, Health and Sexuality* 10,
no. 6 (2008): 556.

P. 155 J. Adams, "Japan: Nothing Says Springtime
like Penis and Vagina Festivals," http://www
.globalpost.com/dispatch/japan/100315/
japan-penis-japanese-vaginas (accessed 20
December 2010).

To Love and Learn

P. 157 Cameron, "Desert Woman," *Canadian
Woman Studies* 26, no. 3–4 (2008): 20.

BIBLIOGRAPHY

"About Endometriosis." http://www.endome
triosis.org/endometriosis.html (accessed 15
September 2008).

Adams, J. "Japan: Nothing Says Springtime like
Penis and Vagina Festivals." http://www.global-
post.com/dispatch/japan/100315
/japan-penis-japanese-vaginas (20 December 2010).

Adams, J. A., A. S. Botash, and N. Kellogg. "Differences in Hymenal Morphology between
Adolescent Girls with and without a History
of Consensual Sexual Intercourse." *Archives of
Pediatrics and Adolescent Medicine* 158, no. 3
(2004): 280–85.

Addiego, F., E. G. Belzer Jr., J. Comolli, W. Moger,
J. D. Perry, and B. Whipple. "Female Ejaculation:
A Case Study." *The Journal of Sex Research* 17,
no. 1 (1981): 13–21.

American Association of Retired Persons. "Attitudes about Sexuality and Aging." *Sexuality in
Midlife and Beyond* (2007): 11–12. http://www
.aarp.org/health/conditions/articles/harvard
_sexuality-in-midlife-and-beyond_2.html (accessed 27 July 2009).

American Nurses Association. "Menopausal
Health: An Overview and Short-Term Benefits
of Hormone Replacement Therapy." http://
www.nursingworld.org/mods/archive/mod130
/cemharef.htm#54 (accessed 6 July 2009).

Amsel, R., P. A. Totten, C. A. Spiegel, K. C. Chen,
D. Eschenbach, and K. K. Holmes. "Nonspecific
Vaginitis: Diagnostic Criteria and Microbial and
Epidemiologic Associations." *American Journal
of Medicine* 74, no. 1 (1983): 14–22.

Amuzu, B. J. "Nonsurgical Therapies for Urinary
Incontinence." *Clinical Obstetrics and Gynecology* 41, no. 3 (1998): 702–11.

Amy, J. "Certificates of Virginity and Reconstruction of the Hymen." *The European Journal of
Contraception and Reproductive Health Care* 13,
no. 2 (2008): 111–13.

"Anal Bleaching." http://bestanalbleaching.com
(accessed 14 March 2008).

Anderson, S. E., G. E. Dallal, and A. Must. "Relative
Weight and Race Influence Average Age at
Menarche: Results from Two Nationally Repre-
sentative Surveys of US Girls Studied 25 Years
Apart." *Pediatrics* 111, no. 4 (2003): 844–50.

"Andre Maurois Quotes." http://www.brainyquote
.com/quotes/quotes/a/andremauro158002.
html (accessed 22 July 2009).

Anitei, S. "New Perfumes Smell Like Sweat, Blood,
Saliva and Sperm." http://news.softpedia.com
(accessed 14 November 2008).

Armstrong, M. L., J. R. Koch, J. C. Saunders, A. E. Roberts, and D. C. Owen. "The Hole Picture: Risks, Decision Making, Purpose, Regulations, and the Future of Body Piercing." *Clinics in Dermatology* 25, no. 4 (2007): 398–406.

AVERT. "Aids Orphans." http://www.avert.org /aids-orphans.htm (accessed 15 September 2009).

AVERT. "Condoms: History, Testing Effectiveness and Availability." http://www.avert.org/con doms.htm (accessed 2 June 2009).

Ayikukwei, R., D. Ngare, J. Sidle, D. Ayuku, J. Balid- dawa, and J. Greene. "HIV/AIDS and Cultural Practices in Western Kenya: The Impact of Sexual Cleansing Rituals on Sexual Behaviours." *Culture, Health and Sexuality* 10, no. 6 (2008): 587–99.

Bagnol, B., and E. Mariano. "Vaginal Practices: Eroticism and Implications for Women's Health and Condom Use in Mozambique." *Culture, Health and Sexuality* 10, no. 6 (2008): 573–85.

Baker, R. R., and M. A. Bellis. "Human Sperm Competition: Ejaculate Adjustment by Males and the Function of Masturbation." *Animal Behaviour* 46, no. 5 (1993): 861–85.

Basnayake, S. "The Virginity Test: a Bridal Night- mare." *Journal of Family Welfare* 36, no. 2 (1990): 50–59.

Batchelor, J. *John Ruskin: A Life.* New York: Carroll & Graf Publishers, 2000.

Beckman, N., M. Waem, D. Gustafson, and I. Skoog. "Secular Trends in Self-Reported Sexual Activity and Satisfaction in Swedish 70-Year- Olds: Cross-Sectional Survey of Four Popu- lations, 1971–2001." *British Medical Journal* 337, no. 7662 (2008): 151–55.

Berensen, A., A. Heger, J. Hayes, R. Bailey, and S. Emans. "Appearance of the Hymen in Pre- pubertal Girls." *Pediatrics* 89 (1992): 387–95.

Betts, H. "Let Us Spray." *The Guardian*, 6 December 2008. http://www.guardian.co.uk (accessed 26 April 2008).

Blackledge, C. "Vaginas, Les Cons, Weather-mak- ers, and Palaces of Delight: Experts from The Story of the V: A Natural History of Female Sexuality." In *Everything You Know about Sex Is Wrong: The Disinformation Guide to the Ex- tremes of Human Sexuality, and Everything in Between,* edited by R. Kick, 268–270. New York: The Disinformation Company, 2006.

Blackledge, C. *The Story of V: A Natural History of Female Sexuality.* New Jersey: Rutgers Univer- sity Press, 2003.

Blinn Pike, L. "Sexuality and Your Child: For Chil- dren Ages 3 to 7." http://extension.missouri.edu /publications/DisplayPub.aspx?P=GH6002 (accessed 13 May 2008).

Boikanyo, E. "So Much for Women-Sensitive Sexual Relations: The Use of Vaginal Potions." *Women and Health* 15 (1992): 4.

Boskey, E. "What Should I Know about the Hymen?" http://std.about.com/od/stdsinthe media/f/hymenfaq.htm (accessed 7 June 2007).

Bradshaw, C. S., A. N. Morton, J. Hocking, S. M. Garland, M. B. Morris, L. M. Moss, L. B. Horvath, I. Kuzevska, and C. K. Fairley. "High Recurrence Rates of Bacterial Vaginosis over the Course of 12 Months after Oral Metronidazole Therapy and Factors Associated with Recurrence." *Journal of Infectious Diseases* 193, no. 11 (2006): 1478–86.

Braun, S. "Labial Trim." http://www.drbraun.co.za /plastic-surgery-procedures/labial-trim.htm (accessed 27 January 2009).

Braun, V., and C. Kitzinger. "Snatch, Hole, or Honey-Pot? Semantic Categories and the Problem of Nonspecificity in Female Genital Slang." *Journal of Sex Research* 38, no. 2 (2001): 146–58.

Braunstein, S., and J. van de Wijgert. *Cultural Norms and Behavior Regarding Vaginal Lubrication During Sex: Implications for the Acceptability of Vaginal Microbicides for the Prevention of HIV/STIs*. New York: The Population Council, 2003.

Brewer, D. J., and E. Teeter. *Ancient Egyptian Society and Family Life*. Cambridge, UK: Cambridge University Press, 2001. http://www.fathom.com /course/21701778/session2.html.

Brulliard, K. "Zulus Eagerly Defy Ban on Virginity Test: South Africa's Progressive Constitution Collides with Tribal Customs." *Washington Post*, 26 September 2008. http://www.washington post.com/wp-dyn/content/article/2008/09 /25/AR2008092504625.html (accessed 6 June 2009).

Brzezinski, A., and A. Benshushan. "Estrogen for Vulvovaginal Symptoms: How Low Can You Go?" *The Journal of the North American Menopause Society* 16, no. 5 (2009): 848–50.

Bullough, V. L. "Masturbation: A Historical Overview." *Journal of Psychology and Human Sexuality* 14, no. 2–3 (2002): 17–33.

Burri, A. V., L. Cherkas, and T. D. Spector. "Genetic and Environmental Influences on Self-Reported G-Spots in Women: A Twin Study." *Journal of Sexual Medicine* 7, no. 5 (2010): 1842–52.

Butterfield, J. *Collins Spanish Dictionary*. http:// www.credoreference.com.ez.sun.ac.za/vol/514 (accessed 1 July 2011).

Cameron, J. "Desert Woman." *Canadian Woman Studies* 26, no. 3–4 (2008): 20.

Cardozo, L., G. Bachmann, D. McClish, D. Fonda, L. Birgerson, L. Cardozo, G. Bachmann, D. McClish, D. Fonda, and L. Birgerson. "Meta-analysis of Estrogen Therapy in the Management of Urogenital Atrophy in Postmenopausal Women: Second Report of the Hormones and

Urogenital Therapy Committee." *Obstetrics and Gynecology* 92, no. 4 (1998): 722–27.

Cartwright, R., and L. Cardoza. "Cosmetic Vulvovaginal Surgery." *Obstetrics, Gynaecology and Reproductive Medicine* 18, no. 10 (2006): 285–86.

Castelo-Branco, C., M. J. Cancelo, J. Villero, F. Nohales, and M. D. Juliá. "Management of Post-Menopausal Vaginal Atrophy and Atrophic Vaginitis." *Maturitas* 52, suppl. 1 (2005): 46–52.

Centers for Disease Control and Prevention. "Bacterial Vaginosis: CDC Fact Sheet." http://www.cdc.gov/std/bv/STDFact-Bacterial-Vaginosis.htm#Complications (accessed 2 August 2009).

Centers for Disease Control and Prevention. "Chlamydia: CDC Fact Sheet." http://www.cdc.gov/std/Chlamydia/STDFact-Chlamydia.htm (accessed 26 August 2009).

Centers for Disease Control and Prevention. "Genital Human Papillomavirus: CDC Fact Sheet." http://www.cdc.gov/STD/HPV/STDFact-HPV.htm (accessed 26 August 2009).

Centers for Disease Control and Prevention. "Gonorrhea: CDC Fact Sheet." http://www.cdc.gov/std/Gonorrhea/STDFact-gonorrhea.htm (accessed 27 August 2009).

Centers for Disease Control and Prevention. "Herpes: CDC Fact Sheet." http://www.cdc.gov/std/herpes/STDFact-herpes.htm (accessed 2 August 2009).

Centers for Disease Control and Prevention.

"Human Papillomavirus (HPV) Infection: CDC Fact Sheet." http://www.cdc.gov/std/HPV/STDFact-HPV.htm (accessed 3 August 2009).

Centers for Disease Control and Prevention. "Pelvic Inflammatory Disease: CDC Fact Sheet." http://www.cdc.gov/std/PID/STDFact-PID.htm (accessed 23 August 2009).

Centers for Disease Control and Prevention. "Syphilis: CDC Fact Sheet." http://www.cdc.gov/std/syphilis/syphilis-fact-sheet.pdf (accessed 3 August 2009).

Centers for Disease Control and Prevention. "Trichomoniasis: CDC Fact Sheet." http://www.cdc.gov/std/trichomonas/default.htm (accessed 21 August 2009).

Centers for Disease Control and Prevention. "Vaccines & Immunizations." http://www.cdc.gov/vaccines/vpd-vac/hpv/vac-faqs.htm (accessed 20 August 2009).

Center for Actuarial Research. "The Impact of Aids on Orphanhood in South Africa: A Quantitative Analysis." http://www.commerce.uct.ac.za/Research_Units/CARE/Monographs/Monographs/mono04.pdf (accessed 23 September 2009).

Cheung, A. M., R. Chaudhry, M. Kapral, C. Jackevicius, and G. Robinson. "Perimenopausal and Postmenopausal Health." *BioMed Central (BMC) Women's Health* 4 (2004): S23.

Childbirth Connection. "Cesarean Section: Best

Evidence." http://www.childbirthconnection
.org/article.asp?ck=10166 (accessed 14 June
2009).

Childbirth Connection. "Preventing Pelvic Floor
Dysfunction." http://www.childbirthconnection
.org/article.asp?ClickedLink=281&ck=10206&area
=27 (accessed 9 July 2009).

Choi, H., M. H. Palmer, and J. Park. "Meta-analysis
of Pelvic Floor Muscle Training: Randomized
Controlled Trials in Incontinent Women." *Nursing Research* 56, no. 4 (2007): 226–34.

Chozick, A. "US Women Seek a Second First Time
with Hymen Surgery." *The Wall Street Journal*,
December 2005. http://www.urogyn.org/docu
ments/HymenoplastyonWSJ.doc (accessed 8
June 2009).

Cindoglu, D. "Virginity Tests and Artificial Virginity
in Modern Turkish Medicine." *Women's Studies
International Forum* 20, no. 2 (1997): 253–61.

Clemons, J. L. "Vaginal Pessary Treatment of
Prolapse and Incontinence." http://www.up
todate.com/patients/content/topic.do?topic
Key=~ntj_vEOf1Aek0h (accessed 15 July 2009).

Coleman, E. "Masturbation as a Means of Achieving Sexual Health." *Psychology and Human
Sexuality* 14, no. 2–3 (2002): 5–16.

Comings, D. E., D. Muhleman, J. P Johnson, and J.
P. MacMurray. "Parent–Daughter Transmission
of the Androgen Receptor Gene as an Explanation of the Effect of Father Absence on Age

of Menarche." *Child Development* 73 (2002):
1046–51.

Costos, D., R. Ackerman, and L. Paradis. "Recollections of Menarche: Communication Between
Mothers and Daughters Regarding Menstruation." *Sex Roles* 46, no. 1–2 (2002): 29–59.

Crooks, R., and K. Baur. *Sexual Arousal and Response.* 10th ed. Belmont, CA: Thomson Higher
Education, 2008.

Cudmore, S. L., K. L. Delgaty, S. F. Hayward-Mc-
Clelland, D. P. Petrin, and G. E. Garber.
"Treatment of Infections Caused by Metronidazole-Resistant Trichomonas Vaginalis." *Clinical Microbiology Reviews* 17, no. 4 (2004): 783–93.

Currie, H. *Menopause: Answers at Your Fingertips.*
London: Class Publishing, 2006.

Darling, C. A., J. K. Davidson Sr., and C. Conway-Welch. "Female Ejaculation: Perceived
Origins, the Gräfenberg Spot/Area, and Sexual
Responsiveness." *Archives of Sexual Behavior* 19,
no. 1 (1990): 29–47.

Dawson, B. E. *Orificial Surgery: Its Philosophy, Application and Technique.* Newark, NJ: The Physician's Drug News Co., 1912.

Deeks, A. A., and M. P. McCabe. "Well-being and
Menopause: An Investigation of Purpose in
Life, Self-Acceptance and Social Role in Premenopausal, Perimenopausal and Postmenopausal Women." *Quality of Life Research* 13, no. 2
(2004): 389–98.

De Havilland, N. "Girls' Virginity Testing an Assault on Human Rights?" *ConsWatch* 1, no. 2 (2007): 2–9.

Delvin, D., and C. Webber. "The G-Spot." http://www.netdoctor.co.uk/healthyliving/gspot.htm (accessed 19 August 2008).

DeMello, M. *Encyclopedia of Body Adornment.* Westport, CT: Greenwood Press, 2007.

Dennerstein, L., P. Lehert, J. R. Guthrie, and H. G. Burger. "Modeling Women's Health During the Menopausal Transition: A Longitudinal Analysis." *The Journal of the North American Menopause Society* 14, no. 1 (2006): 53–62.

Dennerstein, L., A. M. A. Smith, C. A. Morse, and H. G. Burger. "Sexuality and the Menopause." *Journal of Psychosomatic Obstetrics and Gynecology* 15, no. 1 (1994): 59–66. http://www.informaworld.com.ez.sun.ac.za/smpp/title~db=all~content=t713634100~tab=issueslist~branches=15 - v15.

"Djibouti's Women Fight Mutilation." *Mail and Guardian*, July 2005. http://www.mg.co.za/article/2005-07-12-djiboutis-women-fight-mutilation (accessed 12 April 2009).

Dokovska, N. "Hymen Repair Surgery in Macedonia: A Virgin Again for 400 Euros." http://www.thewip.net/contributors/2007/07/hymen_repair_surgery_in_macedo.html (accessed 18 May 2009).

Donald, M., J. Lucke, M. Dunne, and B. Raphael. "Gender Differences Associated with Young People's Emotional Reactions to Sexual Intercourse." *Journal of Youth and Adolescence* 24, no. 4 (1995): 453–64.

Douki, S., B. S. Zineb, F. Nacef, and U. Halbreich. "Women's Mental Health in the Muslim World: Cultural, Religious, and Social Issues." *Journal of Affective Disorders* 102, no. 1 (2007): 177–89.

Drenth, J. *The Origin of the World: Science and Fiction of the Vagina.* Translated by Arnold and Erica Pomerans. London: Reaction Books, 2005.

Driggs, D., and K. Risch. *Hot Pink: The Girls' Guide to Primping, Passion, and Pubic Fashion.* http://ebooks.ebookmall.com/ebook/117270-ebook.htm (accessed 14 November 2009).

Dunne, E. F., E. R. Unger, M. Sternberg, G. McQuillan, D. C. Swan, S. S. Patel, and L. E. Markowitz. "Prevalence of HPV Infection among Females in the United States." *Journal of the American Medical Association* 297, no. 8 (2007): 813–19.

Durso, B. "Girls and Puberty." http://www.keepkidshealthy.com/development/puberty_girls.html (accessed 11 June 2009).

Else, L., R. Persaud, and S. Hite. "The Woman Who Dared to Ask." *New Scientist* 166, no. 2242 (2000): 40–43.

Emans, S. J. "Physical Examination of the Child and Adolescent." In *Evaluation of the Sexually Abused Child: A Medical Textbook and Photographic Atlas*, edited by A. H. Heger, S. J. Emans, and D. Muran, 61–65. 2nd ed. New York: Oxford University Press, 2000.

En.Organisasi.Org Community and Library Online. "Vagina in Other Language than English: Online Translation Dictionary." http://en.organisasi.org/translation/vagina-in-other-languages (accessed July 2011).

"Epic of Gilgamesh." http://looklex.com/e.o/gilgamesh.htm (accessed 19 July 2008).

Ericksen Paige, K. "The Ritual of Circumcision." Human Nature 1(5): 40–48.

E-medicine Health. "Vaginal Bleeding." http://www.emedicinehealth.com/vaginal_bleeding/article_em.htm (accessed 7 June 2009).

Ensler, E. The Vagina Monologues: The V-Day Edition. New York: Villard Books, 2008. http://www.scribd.com/doc/30286086/Eve-Ensler-The-Vagina-Monologues (accessed 27 November 2009).

Etymology Dictionary. http://www.etymonline.com (accessed January–November 2009).

"Evolution and Revolution: The Past, Present, and Future of Contraception." Baylor College of Medicine 10, no. 6 (2000). http://www.contraceptiononline.org/contrareport/article01.cfm?art=93 (accessed May 29, 2009).

"FDA Backs New Cervical Cancer Vaccine Cervarix." http://www.msnbc.msn.com/id/32760999/ns/health-sexual_health (accessed 3 October 2009).

Feldman-Jacobs, C., and D. Clifton. "Female Genital Mutilation/Cutting: Data and Trends." 2008. http://www.prb.org/Publications/Datasheets/2008/fgm2008.aspx (accessed 18 November 2008).

"Francisco de Goya Paintings." http://www.paintinghere.com/artist-1/Francisco-de-Goya-Paintings.html (accessed 3 February 2009).

Francoeur, R. T., and R. J. Noonan, eds. The Continuum Complete International Encyclopedia of Sexuality. http://www.kinseyinstitute.org/ccies (accessed 26 July 2009).

Freedman, M., A. M. Kaunitz, K. Z. Reape, H. Hait, and H. Shu. "Twice-Weekly Synthetic Conjugated Estrogens Vaginal Cream for the Treatment of Vaginal Atrophy." The Journal of the North American Menopause Society 16, no. 4 (2009): 735–41.

Ge, X., M. N. Natsuaki, J. M. Neiderhiser, and D. Reiss. "Genetic and Environmental Influences on Pubertal Timing: Results from Two National Sibling Studies." Journal of Research on Adolescence 17, no. 4 (2007): 767–88.

"Genital Piercing." http://www.primalurge.com.au/index.php?id=34 (accessed 18 March 2009).

George, E. R. "Virginity Testing and South Africa's HIV/AIDS Crisis: Beyond Rights, Universalism and Cultural Relativism Toward Health Capabilities." Californian Law Review 96, no. 6 (2008): 1447–1519.

Gerressu, M., C. H. Mercer, C. A. Graham, K. Wellings, and A. M. Johnson. "Prevalence of Masturbation and Associated Factors in a British National Probability Survey." *Archives of Sexual Behavior* 37, no. 2 (2008): 266–78.

Gibbs, R. S. "Asymptomatic Bacterial Vaginosis: Is It Time to Treat?" *American Journal of Obstetrics and Gynecology* 196, no. 6 (2007): 495–96.

Giblin, K. L. "Sex and Menopause: The Sizzle and the Fizzle." *Sexuality, Reproduction and Menopause* 3, no. 2 (2005): 72–77.

Ginsberg, J. "What Determines the Age at the Menopause?" *British Medical Journal* 302, no. 6788 (1991): 1288–89.

Ginway, M. E. *Brazilian Science Fiction: Cultural Myths and Nationhood in the Land of the Future.* Cranbury, NJ: Associated University Press, 2004.

Gita, D. M., W. J. Brown, and A. J. Dobson. "Physical and Mental Health: Changes During Menopause Transition." *Quality of Life Research* 12 (2003): 405–12.

Glenville, M. "Prolapse." http://www.marilynglenville.com/general/prolapse.htm (accessed 27 July 2009).

Golingai, P. "Pressure for Pleasure." *Malaysian Star*, 5 March 2006. http://thestar.com.my/lifestyle/story.asp?file=/2006/3/5/lifefocus/13553248&sec=lifefocus (accessed 16 March 2009).

Google. "Google Translate." http://translate.google.com/?hl=af# (accessed September 2009).

Gordon, B. N., and C. S. Schroeder. *Sexuality: A Developmental Approach to Problems.* New York: Plenum Press, 1995.

Graber, C. "Strange but True: Whale Waste Is Extremely Valuable." http://www.scientificamerican.com/article.cfm?id=strange-but-true-whale-waste-is-valuable (accessed 6 March 2012).

Gräfenberg, E. "The Role of Urethra in Female Orgasm." *International Journal of Sexology* 3, no. 3 (1950): 145–48.

Gravina, G. L., F. Brandetti, P. Martini, E. Carosa, S. M. Di Stasi, S. Morano, A. Lenzi, and E. A. Jannini. "Measurement of the Thickness of the Urethrovaginal Space in Women with or without Vaginal Orgasm." *Journal of Sexual Medicine* 5, no. 3 (2008): 610–18.

Green, F. J. "From Clitoridectomies to 'Designer Vaginas': The Medical Construction of Heteronormative Female Bodies and Sexuality Through Female Genital Cutting." *Sexualities, Evolution and Gender* 7, no. 2 (2005): 153–87.

Hamilton, T. *Skin Flutes and Velvet Gloves: A Collection of Facts and Fancies, Legends and Oddities about the Body's Private Parts.* New York: St. Martin's Press, 2002.

Herdt, G. H., ed. *Ritualized Homosexuality in Melanesia.* Berkeley: University of California Press, 1993.

Hales, D. *An Invitation to Health.* Belmont, CA: Cengage Learning. http://www.cengagebrain

.com/shop/content/hales88556_0495388556_01.01_toc.pdf (accessed January 2011).

Hall, P. "Sexual Health: Enjoying Sex." http://www.bbc.co.uk/relationships/sex_and_sexual_health/enjsex_gspot.shtml (accessed 18 July 2009).

Hallfors, D. D., M. W. Waller, C. A. Ford, C. T. Halpern, P. H. Brodish, and B. Iritani. "Adolescent Depression and Suicide Risk: Association with Sex and Drug Behavior." *American Journal of Preventive Medicine* 27, no. 3 (2004): 224–31.

Hamilton, T. *Skin Flutes and Velvet Gloves: A Collection of Facts and Fancies, Legends and Oddities about the Body's Private Parts*. New York: St. Martin's Press, 2002.

Handa, V. L. "Sexual Function and Childbirth." *Seminars in Perinatology* 30, no. 5 (2006): 253–56.

Hannestad, Y. S., G. Rortveit, H. Sandvik, and S. A. Hunskaar. "A Community-based Epidemiological Survey of Female Urinary Incontinence: Norwegian EPINCONT Study — Epidemiology of Incontinence, the Nord-Trøndelag Health Survey." *Journal of Clinical Epidemiology* 53 (2000): 1150–57.

Hansen, L., J. Mann, S. McMahon, and T. Wong. "Sexual Health." *BioMed Central (BMC) Women's Health* 4, suppl. 1 (2004): S24.

HarperCollins. *Collins English-Polish Dictionary.*

http://www.credoreference.com.ez.sun.ac.za/book/collinsengpol (accessed 22 June 2011).

HarperCollins. *Collins Essential Thesaurus*. http://www.thefreedictionary.com/_/misc/HarperCollinsProducts.aspx?EnglishThesaurus (accessed January–November 2009).

HarperCollins. *Collins French Dictionary Plus.* http://www.credoreference.com.ez.sun.ac.za/vol/503 (accessed 22 June 2011).

HarperCollins. *Collins German Dictionary*. http://www.credoreference.com.ez.sun.ac.za/vol/529 (accessed 23 June 2011).

HarperCollins. *Collins Italian Dictionary*. http://www.credoreference.com.ez.sun.ac.za/vol/511 (accessed 22 June 2011).

Harvard Health Publications "Atrophic Vaginitis." http://www.health.harvard.edu/newsletters/Harvard_Womens_Health_Watch (accessed 14 April 2009).

Hemminki, E., P. Veerus, H. Pisarev, S. Hovi, P. Topo, and H. Karro. "The Effects of Postmenopausal Hormone Therapy on Social Activity, Partner Relationship, and Sexual Life: Experience from the EPHT Trial." *BioMed Central (BMC) Women's Health* 9 (2009): 16.

Henderson, V. W. "Memory at Midlife: Perception and Misperception." *The Journal of the North American Menopause Society* 16, no. 4 (2009): 635–36.

Henna Body Art. "Henna and Mehndi Tattoos: Where It All Started and Why." http://www.henna-tattoos-kits.com/henna-tattoo/history.htm (accessed 14 March 2009).

Hesse, W. R. Jr. *Jewelry Making Through World History: An Encyclopedia.* London: Greenwood Press, 2007.

Hilton, T. *John Ruskin.* New Haven, CT: Yale University Press, 2002.

Hines, T. "The G-Spot: A Modern Gynecologic Myth." *American Journal of Obstetrics and Gynecology* 185, no. 2 (2002): 359–62.

Hitti, M. "Sex after 70 Getting Better: Swedish Study." http://www.webmd.com/sex-relationships/news/20080708/sex-after-70-better-than-in-the-past (accessed 19 July 2009).

Hlongwa, W. "Girls Flock to Get Virginity Certificate." *The Mercury,* 23 August 1999. http://www.themercury.co.za (accessed 27 March 2009).

Hobday, A. J., L. Haury, and P. K. Dayton. "Function of the Human Hymen." *Medical Hypotheses* 49, no. 2 (1997): 171–73.

Hoby, H. "The Fashion Designer Mary Quant." *The Guardian,* 21 June 2009. http://www.guardian.co.uk/society/2009/jun/21/older-people-fashion-designers (accessed 23 August 2009).

ILGA (International Lesbian, Gay, Bisexual, Trans and Intersex Association) "World Day Against Death Penalty." http://ilga.org/ilga/en/article/1111 (accessed 24 August 2011).

"Incontinence Overview, Incidence and Prevalence of Urinary Incontinence." http://www.urologychannel.com/incontinence/index.shtml (accessed 5 July 2008).

"Indigenous People of the Amazon Native Amazonian Tribe." http://www.matses.info (accessed 10 February 2009).

Isa, A. R., R. Shuib, and M. Shukri Othman. "The Practice of Female Circumcision among Muslims in Kelantan, Malaysia." *Reproductive Health Matters* 7 (May 1999): 137–44.

Jamieson, L., and P. Proudlock. "Children's Bill Progress." http://web.uct.ac.za/depts/ci/plr/cbill.htm (accessed 14 May 2009).

Jayne, C. "The Dark Continent Revisited: An Examination of the Freudian View of Female Orgasm." *Psychoanalysis and Contemporary Thought* 3 (1980): 545–68.

Johnson, J. "Exposed at Last: The Truth about Your Clitoris." *Herizons: The Manitoba Women's Newspaper* 12, no. 3 (1998): 19–21.

Joint United Nations Programme on HIV/AIDS. "AIDS Epidemic Update." http://data.unaids.org/pub/EPISlides/2007/2007_epiupdate_en.pdf (accessed 15 September 2009).

Joint United Nations Programme on HIV/AIDS. "2008 Report on the Global AIDS Epidemic: Executive Summary." http://data.unaids.org/pub/GlobalReport/2008/JC1511_GR08_Executive-Summary_en.pdf (accessed 15 September 2009).

Kadri, N., S. Berrada, K. Alami, F. Manoudi, L. Rachidi, S. Maftouh, and U. Halbreich. "Mental Health of Moroccan Women: A Sexual Perspective." *Journal of Affective Disorders* 102, no. 1–3 (2007): 199–207.

Kallings, L. O. "The First Postmodern Pandemic: 25 Years of HIV/AIDS." *Journal of Internal Medicine* 263, no. 3 (2008): 218–43.

Kaufman, D. W., D. Slone, L. Rosenberg, O. S. Miettinen, and S. Shapiro. "Cigarette Smoking and Age at Natural Menopause." *American Journal of Public Health* 70, no. 4 (1980): 420–22.

Kazandjieva, J., I. Grozdev, and N. Tsankov. "Temporary Henna Tattoos." *Clinics in Dermatology* 25, no. 4 (2007): 383–87.

Kazandjieva, J., and N. Tsankov. "Tattoos and Piercings." *Clinics in Dermatology* 25, no. 4 (2007a): 361.

Kazandjieva, J., and N. Tsankov. "Tattoos: Dermatological Complications." *Clinics in Dermatology* 25, no. 4 (2007b): 375–82.

Kelley, C. "Estrogen and Its Effect on Vaginal Atrophy in Post-Menopausal Women." *Urologic Nursing* 27, no. 1 (2007): 40–45.

Kellogg, J. H. "Plain Facts for Old and Young: Embracing History and Hygiene of Organic Life." http://www.gutenberg.org/etext/19924 (accessed 15 May 2009).

Kellogg, J. H. *The Ladies' Guide in Health and Disease*. London: International Tract Society, 1894.

Kellogg, J. H. *Man the Masterpiece*. London: Henry Camp and Co., 1903.

Kellogg, N. D., S. W. Menard, and A. Santos. "Genital Anatomy in Pregnant Adolescents: 'Normal' Does Not Mean 'Nothing Happened.'" *Pediatrics* 113, no. 1 (2004): e67–e69.

Kick, R., ed. *Everything You Know about Sex Is Wrong: The Disinformation Guide to the Extremes of Human Sexuality, and Everything in Between*. New York: The Disinformation Company, 2006.

KidsHealth. "Female Reproductive System." http://kidshealth.org/parent/general/body_basics/female_reproductive_system.html (accessed 15 September 2009).

Kingsley, D. "Early Menopause Is Strongly Genetic." http://www.abc.net.au/science/articles/2001/08/30/354928.htm (accessed 19 July 2009).

Kirsch, R. "Body Piercing: Stick It Where the Sun Don't Shine. The Ups and Downs of Putting Something In." *The McGill Tribune*, 1 November 2000. http://media.www.mcgilltribune.com/media/storage/paper234/news/2000/10/31/Features/Body-Piercing.Stick.It.Where.The.Sun.Don8217t.Shine-7456-page1.shtml (accessed 21 February 2000).

Kitzinger, S. *Woman's Experience of Sex*. Johannesburg, SA: Flower Press, 1985.

Kobrin, S. "US Health: More Women Seek Vaginal

Plastic Surgery." http://www.womensenews
.org/article.cfm/dyn/aid/2067/context/archive
(accessed 14 June 2005).

Koenig, L. M. "Body Piercing: Medical Concerns
with Cutting-Edge Fashion." *Journal of General
Internal Medicine* 14, no. 6 (1999): 379–85.

Kogos, F. *A Dictionary of Yiddish Slang and Idioms.*
New York: Citadel Press, 1995.

Kohl, J. V., and R. T. Francoeur. *The Scent of Eros:
Mysteries of Odor in Human Sexuality.* Lincoln,
NE: iUniverse, 2002.

Kuukasjärvi, S., C. J. P. Eriksson, E. Koskela, T.
Mappes, K. Nissinen, and M. J. Rantala. "Attractiveness of Women's Body Odors over the
Menstrual Cycle: The Role of Oral Contraceptives and Receiver Sex." *Behavioural Ecology* 15,
no. 4 (2004): 579–84.

"Labiaplasty: Cosmetic Vaginal Surgery: Vagino-
plasty (Tightening)." http://www.lasertreat
ments.com/labiaplasty.html (accessed 6
March 2009).

"Labium." http://www.absoluteastronomy.com
/topics/Labium (accessed 18 March 2009).

Lalwani, S., R. H. Reindollar, and A. J. Davis. "Normal Onset of Puberty: Have Definitions of Onset Changed?" *Obstetrics and Gynecology Clinics
of North America* 30, no. 2 (2003): 279–86.

Larsson, I. "Sexual Abuse of Children: Child Sexuality and Sexual Behaviour." Translated by Lambert and Tudball. http://www.childcentre.info
/research/abusedchil/acf6d9.pdf (accessed 7
May 2009).

Larue, G. A. "Ancient Ethics." In *A Companion to
Ethics.* Edited by P. Singer, 29–42. Oxford, UK:
Blackwell Publishing, 1993.

Laser Vaginal Rejuvenation Institute of Michigan.
"Vaginal Rejuvenation: Designer Laser Vagino-
plasty for Aesthetic Surgical Enhancement."
http://www.drberenholz.com (accessed 24
May 2009).

Lee, J. M., D. Appugliese, N. Kaciroti, R. F. Corwyn,
R. H. Bradley, and J. C. Lumeng. "Weight Status
in Young Girls and the Onset of Puberty." *Pediatrics* 119, no. 3 (2007): 593–94.

Lefkowitz, M. R., and M. B. Fant, eds. *Women's Life
in Greece and Rome: A Source Book in Translation.* 2nd ed. Baltimore, MD: Johns Hopkins
University Press, 1992.

Leplège, A., and L. Dennerstein. "Menopause and
Quality of Life." *Quality of Life Research* 9, suppl.
1 (2000): 689–92.

Le Roux, L. "Harmful Traditional Practices: Male
Circumcision and Virginity Testing of Girls and
the Legal Rights of Children." University of the
Western Cape, South Africa, 2006. http://etd
.uwc.ac.za/usrfiles/modules/etd/docs/etd
_gen8Srv25Nme4_8182_1183427422.pdf (accessed 5 February 2009).

Levy, J. *Tattoos in Modern Society.* New York:
Rosen Publishing Group, 2009.

Lewnes, A., ed. "Changing a Harmful Social Convention: Female Genital Mutilation/Cutting." http://www.unicef-irc.org/publications/pdf/fgm_eng.pdf (accessed 27 February 2009).

"Liaisons Dangereuses by Kilian Typical Me." http://fortheloveofperfume.blogspot.com/2007/11/liaisons-dangereuses-by-kilian-typical.html (accessed 8 April 2009).

Lightfoot-Klein, H. "Prisoners of Ritual: Some Contemporary Developments in the History of FGM." http://www.fgmnetwork.org/Lightfoot-klein/prisonersofritual.htm (accessed 5 February 2008).

Maguire, L. "Virginity Tests." http://www.answers.com/topic/virginity-tests (accessed 24 February 2009).

Maines, R. P. *The Technology of Orgasm: "Hysteria," the Vibrator, and Women's Sexual Satisfaction.* Baltimore, MD: The Johns Hopkins University Press, 1998.

Maines, R. P. "Freud and the Steam-Powered Vibrator." In *Longing: Psychoanalytic Musings on Desire.* Edited by J. Petrucelli, 21–138. London: H. Karnac Books, 2006.

Makhlouf Obermeyer, C. "Female Genital Surgeries: The Known, the Unknown, and the Unknowable." *Medical Anthropology Quarterly* 13, no. 1 (1999): 79–106.

Malloy, D. "Body and Genital Piercing in Brief." http://www.bmezine.com/news/jimward/20040315-p.html (accessed 13 February 2009).

Mascall, S. "Time for Rethink on the Clitoris." http://news.bbc.co.uk/1/hi/health/5013866.stm (accessed 11 February 2006).

Mayo Clinic. "Kegel Exercises: A How-To Guide for Women." http://www.mayoclinic.com/health/kegel-exercises/WO00119 (accessed 26 January 2009).

Mazumdar, M. D. "The Cervical Cycle." http://www.gynaeonline.com/cervical_cycle.htm (accessed 23 August 2009).

Mazumbar, M. D. "Vaginal Discharge Without Itching." http://www.gynaeonline.com/vaginitis.htm (accessed 11 August 2009).

McCormack, D. "All in a Stink about Perfume." http://www2.canada.com (accessed 15 April 2009).

McGreal, C. "Virgin Tests Make a Comeback." *Daily Mail & Guardian*, 29 September 1999. http://www.hartford-hwp.com/archives/37a/162.html (accessed 14 June 2009).

McKenna, P. "Childhood Obesity Brings Early Puberty for Girls." http://www.newscientist.com/article/dn11307-childhood-obesity-brings-early-puberty-for-girls.html (accessed 18 June 2009).

Medical Advisory Secretariat. "Midurethral Slings for Women with Stress Urinary Incontinence:

An Evidence-based Analysis." *Ontario Health Technology Assessment Series* 6, no. 3 (2006): 1–61.

MedicineNet.com. "Pelvic Inflammatory Disease." http://www.medicinenet.com/pelvic_inflammatory_disease/article.htm (accessed 3 October 2009).

Medical News Today. "FDA Advisory Committee Makes Favorable Recommendation for Cervarix, GlaxoSmithKline's Candidate Cervical Cancer Vaccine." http://www.medicalnewstoday.com/articles/163453.php (accessed 3 October 2009).

Medical News Today. "Tattoo, Piercing and Breast Implantation Infections." http://www.medicalnewstoday.com/articles/41238.php (accessed 14 March 2009).

MedicineNet.com. "Pubic Lice (Crabs)." http://www.medicinenet.com/pubic_lice_crabs/article.htm (accessed 4 October 2009).

Medicine.Net.com. "Scabies: Symptoms, Signs, Treatments and Facts." http://www.medicinenet.com/scabies/page3.htm (accessed 27 September 2009).

MedlinePlus. "Atrophic Vaginitis." http://www.nlm.nih.gov/medlineplus/ency/article/000892.htm (accessed 3 July 2009).

MedlinePlus. "Chancroid." http://www.nlm.nih.gov/medlineplus/ency/article/000635.htm (accessed 25 October 2009).

Melby, T. "Childhood Sexuality." *Contemporary Sexuality* 35, no. 12 (2001).

MedlinePlus. "Vaginal Discharge." http://www.nlm.nih.gov/medlineplus/ency/article/003158.htm (accessed 14 August 2009).

MedlinePlus. "Vaginal Yeast Infection." http://www.nlm.nih.gov/medlineplus/ency/article/001511.htm (accessed 14 August 2009).

Melby, T. "Childhood Sexuality." *Contemporary Sexuality* 35, no. 12 (2001): 3.

"Menarche." http://www.absoluteastronomy.com/topics/Menarche (accessed 18 August 2009).

Mendle, J., E. Turkheimer, B. M. D'Onofrio, S. K. Lynch, R. E. Emery, W. S. Slutske, and N. G. Martin. "Family Structure and Age at Menarche: A Children-of-Twins Approach." *Developmental Psychology* 42, no. 3 (2006): 533–42.

MERCK. "Chancroid: Sexually Transmitted Diseases." http://www.merck.com/mmpe/sec14/ch194/ch194b.html (accessed 26 October 2009).

Menopause Matters. "Wake up to Sex at 50!" http://www.menopausematters.co.uk/magazinearticle2.php (accessed 14 July 2009).

Merriam Webster Online Dictionary. http://www.merriam-webster.com/ (accessed January–November 2009).

Meston, C. M. "Aging and Sexuality." *Western Journal of Medicine* 167, no. 4 (1997): 285–90.

Micale, M. S. "The Decline of 'Hysteria.'" *Harvard Mental Health Letter* 17, no. 1 (2000): 1–4.

Miranda, C. "The Vagina Dialogue." *Time Magazine*, 29 September 2006. http://www.time.com/time/arts/article/0,8599,1541053,00.html (accessed 20 January 2009).

Morgan-Mar, D. "Australian Aboriginal Magic." http://www.sjgames.com/pyramid/sample.html?id=4291 (accessed 9 June 2008).

Morrison, C. "Body Piercing History." http://www.painfulpleasures.com/piercing_history.htm (accessed 23 February 2008).

Mshana, G., M. L. Plummer, J. Wamoyi, Z. S. Shigongo, D. A. Ross, and D. Wight. "She Was Bewitched and Caught an Illness Similar to AIDS: AIDS and Sexually Transmitted Infection Causation Beliefs in Rural Northern Tanzania." *Culture, Health and Sexuality* 8, no. 1 (2006): 45–52.

Müftüler-Bac, M. "Turkish Women's Predicament: A Short History." *Women's Studies International Forum* 22, no. 3 (1999): 303–15.

Mustanski, B. S., R. J. Viken, J. Kaprio, L. Pulkkinen, and R. J. Rose. "Genetic and Environmental Influences on Pubertal Development: Longitudinal Data from Finnish Twins at Ages 11 and 14." *Developmental Psychology* 40, no. 6 (2004): 1188–98.

Nahid, T. "Female Circumcision as a Public Health Issue." *The New England Journal of Medicine* 331 (1994): 712–16.

Nappi, R., G. Liekens, and U. Brandenburg. "Attitudes, Perceptions and Knowledge about the Vagina: The International Vagina Dialogue Survey." *Contraception* 73, no. 5 (2006): 493–500.

National Cancer Institute. "Menopausal Hormone Replacement Therapy Use and Cancer." http://www.cancernet.gov/cancertopics/factsheet/Risk/menopausal-hormones (accessed 26 July 2009).

National Institute of Allergy and Infectious Diseases. "Workshop Summary: Scientific Evidence on Condom Effectiveness for Sexually Transmitted Disease (STD)." http://www3.niaid.nih.gov/about/organization/dmid/PDF/condomReport.pdf (accessed 29 June 2009).

Newton Long, Q. "Abnormal Vaginal Bleeding." In *Gynecology Principles and Practice*. Edited by R. E. Kirstner, 810–812. 3rd ed. Chicago, IL: Book Medical Publishers, 1979.

Ngalwa, S. "Reed Dance Maidens Back Virginity Testing." *Sunday Tribune*, 11 September 2005. http://www.iol.co.za/index.php?set_id=1&click_id=13&art_id=vn20050911103318938C380876 (accessed 2 June 2009).

Nguyen, J. K., and N. N. Bhatia. "Resolution of Motor Urge Incontinence after Surgical Repair of Pelvic Organ Prolapse." *Journal of Urology* 166, no. 6 (2001): 2263–66.

Nissl, J. "Object in the Vagina." http://health.msn

.com/health-topics/articlepage.aspx?cp-docu
mentid=100078649 (accessed 27 May 2009).

North American Menopause Society. "The Role
of Local Vaginal Estrogen for Treatment of
Vaginal Atrophy in Postmenopausal Women:
Position Statement." *Menopause: The Journal of
the North American Menopause Society* 14, no. 3
(2007): 357–69.

Nottingham, V. "History of Female Contraception."
http://www.medhunters.com/articles/history
OfFemaleContraception.html (accessed 16
January 2009).

Nwosu, E. C., S. Rao, C. Igweike, and H. Hamed.
"Foreign Objects of Long Duration in the Adult
Vagina." *Journal of Obstetrics and Gynaecology*
25, no. 7 (2005): 737–39.

O'Hanlan, K. "Alternative Treatments for Menopausal Symptoms." http://www.ohanlan.com
/PDFs/Alternatives_to_estrogen.pdf (accessed
25 July 2009).

Olesen, A. L., V. J. Smith, J. O. Bergstrom, J. C.
Colling, and A. L. Clark. "Epidemiology of Surgically Managed Pelvic Organ Prolapse and Urinary Incontinence." *Obstetrics and Gynecology*
89, no. 4 (1997): 501–506.

Opie, I., and P. Opie. *The Oxford Dictionary of Nursery Rhymes.* 2nd ed. Oxford: Oxford University
Press, 1997.

"Orificial Surgery: The Orificial Surgery Society
and Orthodox Medicine." http://www.history

ofcircumcision.net/index.php?option=com
_content&task=view&id=52&Itemid=0 (ac-
cessed 18 November 2009).

Paige, K. E. "The Ritual of Circumcision." *Human
Nature* 1, no. 5 (1978): 40–48.

Pantone, D. J. "The Matis and Matsés Indians of
the Amazon Rainforest." http://www.amazon
-indians.org/page02.html (accessed 27 June
2009).

Pappas, P. G. "Invasive Candidiasis." *Infectious Disease Clinics of North America* 20, no. 3 (2006):
485–506.

Pascarl, J. "An Open Letter to Men with Fast Cars
and Fancy Watches." http://www.thepunch
.com.au/articles/an-open-letter-to-middle
-aged-men-with-fast-cars (accessed 15 July
2009).

Pauline, M. "Menopause and Anxiety: Immediate
and Long-Term Effects." *The Journal of the North
American Menopause Society* 15, no. 6 (2008):
1033–35.

Petrucelli, J. *Longing: Psychoanalytic Musings on
Desire.* London: H. Karnac Books, 2006.

Phillips, C., and A. Monga. "Childbirth and the Pelvic Floor: The Gynaecological Consequences."
Reviews in Gynaecological Practice 5, no. 1
(2005): 15–22.

"Physician Offers 'G-Shot' to Enhance Sexual
Function." *Sexual Science* 49, no. 1 (2008): 5.

Pinker, S. *The Stuff of Thought: Language as a*

Window into Human Nature. New York: Penguin Group, 2007.

Planned Parenthood Federation of America. *A History of Birth Control Methods*. New York: Katharine Dexter McCormick Library, 2006. http://www.plannedparenthood.org/files/PPFA/history_bc_methods.pdf (accessed 6 March 2012).

Planned Parenthood Federation of America. "Masturbation: From Myth to Sexual Health." *Contemporary Sexuality* 37, no. 3 (2003): i–vii.

Poniewaz, C. M. "The History of Henna Tattoo Design." http://www.essortment.com/all/historyofhenna_rmfe.htm (accessed 15 March 2008).

Population Reference Bureau. "Female Genital Mutilation/Cutting: Data and Trends." www.prb.org/pdf08/fgm-wallchart.pdf (accessed 24 April 2009).

Primal Urge Piercing. "Genital Piercing." http://www.primalurge.com.au/index.php?id=34 (accessed 18 March 2009).

Quinlan, R. "Father Absence, Parental Care and Female Reproductive Development." *Evolution and Human Behavior* 24, no. 6 (2003): 376–90.

Rector, R. E., K. A. Johnson, and L. R. Noyes. "Sexually Active Teenagers Are More Likely to Be Depressed and to Attempt Suicide." http://www.heritage.org/Research/Family/cda0304.cfm (accessed 30 May 2009).

Ringa, V. "Menopause and Treatments." *Quality of Life Research* 9, no. 6 (2002): 695–707.

Roberts, H. "Reconstructing Virginity in Guatemala." *The Lancet* 367, no. 9518 (2006): 1227–28.

Roberts, H. "Managing the Menopause." *British Medical Journal* 334 (2007): 736–41.

Rockoff, A., and M. C. Stöppler. "Scabies." http://www.medicinenet.com/scabies/article.htm (accessed 27 September 2009).

Rosenbloom, S. "What Did You Call It?" *New York Times*, 28 October 2007. http://www.nytimes.com/2007/10/28/fashion/28vajayjay.html?_r=1&pagewanted=print (accessed 18 January 2009).

Rubin, H. H. *Eugenics and Sex Harmony*. New York: Pioneer Publications, 1938.

Ruscone, L. G. "Sailor Tattoos." http://www.tattoolife.com/archive/arch_16.html (accessed 4 March 2009).

Sample, I. "The Elusive G-Spot Really Does Exist, Say Researchers." *The Guardian UK*, 21 February 2008. http://www.guardian.co.uk/science/2008/feb/21/medicalresearch.sciencenews (accessed 16 September 2009).

Scheinfeld, N. "Tattoos and Religion." *Clinics in Dermatology* 25, no. 4 (2007): 362–66.

Sciolino, E. "In Europe, Debate over Islam and Virginity." *The New York Times*, 11 June 2008. http://www.nytimes.com/2008/06/11/world

/europe/11virgin.html?_r=1 (accessed 28 June 2009).

Sepkowitz, K. A. "AIDS: The First 20 Years." *The New England Journal of Medicine* 344, no. 23 (2001): 1764–73.

"Sex Can Be Better After Menopause." http://www.tidesoflife.com/sexafter.htm (accessed 17 July 2009).

"Sexes: In Search of a Perfect G." *Time Magazine*, 13 September 1982. http://www.time.com/time/magazine/0,9171,951742-1,00.html (accessed 13 September 2009).

"Sexual Response Cycle." http://www.soc.ucsb.edu/sexinfo/article/the-sexual-response-cycle#four (accessed 31 June 2009).

"Sexual Violence Research Initiative (SVRI)." http://www.svri.org (accessed 23 January 2009).

Shalhoub-Kevorkian, N. "Imposition of Virginity Testing: A Life-Saver or a License to Kill?" *Social Science and Medicine* 60, no. 6 (2005): 1187–96.

Sik Ying Ho, P., and A. Ka Tat Tsang. "Beyond the Vagina-Clitoris Debate: From Naming the Genitals to Reclaiming the Woman's Body." *Women's Studies International Forum* 28, no. 6 (2005): 523–34.

Skoll, P. J. "Vaginal Labiaplasty." http://www.plasticsurgeon.co.za (accessed 11 February 2008).

Smith, G. R. Jr. *Somatization Disorder in the Medical Setting*. Washington, DC: American Psychiatric Press, 1991.

South Asian Women's Forum. "Vaginal Surgery, Including 'Revirgination': Newest Trend for US Women." http://www.sawf.org/newedit/edit01162006/news.asp (accessed 16 January 2006).

Steigrad, A. "Muslim Women in France Regain Virginity in Clinics." http://www.alertnet.org/thenews/newsdesk/L25320251.htm (accessed 30 February 2009).

Stengers, J., and A. van Neck. *Masturbation: The History of a Great Terror*. Translated by K. Hoffmann. New York: Palgrave, 2001.

Stern, K., and M. K. McClintock. "Regulation of Ovulation by Human Pheromones." *Nature* 392 (1998): 177–79.

Stöppler, M. C. "Genital Herpes in Women." http://www.medicinenet.com/genital_herpes_in_women/article.htm (accessed 3 August 2009).

Stöppler, M. C. "Gonorrhea in Women." http://www.medicinenet.com/gonorrhea_in_women/article.htm (accessed 25 September 2009).

Stöppler, M. C. "Sexually Transmitted Diseases (STDs) in Women." http://www.medicinenet.com/sexually_transmitted_diseases_stds_in_women/article.htm (accessed 2 August 2009).

Stöppler, M. C. "Syphilis in Women." http://www

.medicinenet.com/syphilis_in_women/page2
.htm (accessed 22 September 2009).

Stöppler, M. C. "Vaginal Bleeding." http://www
.medicinenet.com/vaginal_bleeding/article
.htm (accessed 27 August 2009).

Sundahl, D. *Female Ejaculation & the G-Spot.*
Alameda, CA: Hunter House Publishers, 2003.

Supriya, S. "Celebrating Womanhood." http://liv
ing.oneindia.in/expressions/celebrate-woman
hood.html (accessed 24 May 2008).

Surbey, M. K. "Family Composition, Stress, and the
Timing of Human Menarche." In *Socioendocri-
nology of Primate Reproduction*, edited by T. E.
Ziegler and F. B. Bercovitch, 11–32. New York:
Wiley-Liss, 1990.

Tanner, J. M., and P. S. Davies. "Clinical Longitudinal Standards for Height and Height Velocity
for North American Children." *The Journal of
Pediatrics* 107, no. 3 (1985): 317–29.

Tanner, J. M., and R. H. Whitehouse. "Clinical
Longitudinal Standards for Height, Weight,
Height Velocity, Weight Velocity, and Stages of
Puberty." *Archives in Disease in Children* 51, no. 3
(1976): 170–79.

TeensHealth. "HIV and AIDS." http://kidshealth.org
/teen/sexual_health/stds/std_hiv.html (accessed 5 August 2009).

Teyise, T. "The Cruelest Cut." http://www.health-e
.org.za/news/article.php?uid=20030914 (accessed 18 March 2009).

Thabet, S. M. A. "Reality of the G-Spot and Its
Relation to Female Circumcision and Vaginal
Surgery." *Journal of Obstetrics and Gynaecology
Research* 35, no. 5 (2009): 967–73.

"The History of Jewelry: Ethnic Tribal Jewelry."
http://www.khulsey.com/jewelry/jewelry
_history_primitive_ethnic_tribal.html (accessed 14 January 2009).

"The Hymen." http://www.soc.ucsb.edu/sexinfo
/article/the-hymen (accessed 2 March 2009).

"The Impact of Menopause: Survey Results."
http://www.emaxhealth.com/1/70/32545/im
pact-menopause-survey-results.html (accessed 2 July 2009).

Thiele, A. "Ancient Egyptian Midwifery and
Childbirth." http://www.mnsu.edu/emuseum
/prehistory/egypt/dailylife/midwifery.htm
(accessed 16 November 2008).

Torres, N. "How to Make an Aspirin Mask." http://
hairremoval.about.com/od/shaving/a/aspirin
-mask.htm (accessed 25 February 2009).

Torres, N. "Ingrown Hair Home Treatment." http://
hairremoval.about.com/od/shaving/a/in
grown-home.htm (accessed 25 February 2009).

"Toxic Shock Syndrome." http://www.humpath
.com/toxic-shock-syndrome (accessed 4 August 2009).

Ubillos, S., D. Paez, and J. L. González. "Culture and
Sexual Behavior." *Psicothema* 12 (2000): 70–82.

Uniformed Services University of the Health

Sciences. "Deployment Dermatology." http://rad.usuhs.mil/derm/lecture_notes/Norton_deployderm.htm (accessed 13 October 2009).

United Nations Development Fund for Women. "Violence against Women: Facts and Figures." http://www.unifem.org/attachments/gender_issues/violence_against_women/facts_figures_violence_against_women_2007.pdf (accessed 13 February 2009).

United States Department of Health and Human Services. "National Guideline for the Management of Bacterial Vaginosis." http://www.guideline.gov/index.aspx (accessed 4 August 2009).

University of Maryland Medical Center. "Atrophic Vaginitis: Overview." http://www.umm.edu/ency/article/000892.htm (accessed July 14 2009).

"Vaginal Cosmetic Surgery." http://www.labiaplastysurgeon.com (accessed 26 May 2009).

"Vaginal Yeast Infection." http://www.nlm.nih.gov/medlineplus/ency/article/001511.htm (accessed 14 August 2009).

Van Duynhoven, Y. T. H. P. "The Epidemiology of Neisseria Gonorrhoeae in Europe." Microbes and Infection 1, no. 6 (1999): 455–64.

Van Schoor, J. "Gardasil™: Quadrivalent HPV Vaccine." SA Pharmaceutical Journal 75, no. 4 (2008): 34.

"Virginity Test for Boys on Cards." http://www.news24.com/News24/Archive/0,,2-1659_1137520,00.html (accessed 4 May 2009).

Vulva Original. "Vulva Intimate Perfume." http://www.smellmeand.com/index_2.html %5B20081 (accessed 4 October 2009).

Waetjen, L. E., L. L. Subak, H. Shen, F. Lin, T. H. Wang, E. Vittinghoff, and J. S. Brown. "Stress Urinary Incontinence Surgery in the United States." Obstetrics and Gynecology 101, no. 4 (2003): 671–76.

Waldenström, U. "Normal Childbirth and Evidence-based Practice." Women and Birth 20, no. 4 (2007): 175–80.

Walid, M. S. "Prevalence of Urinary Incontinence in Female Residents of American Nursing Homes and Association with Neuropsychiatric Disorders." Journal of Clinical Medicine Research 1, no. 1 (2009): 37–39.

WebMD. "Sex Glossary." http://www.webmd.com/sexual-conditions/sexual-health-glossary?page=15 (accessed 28 August 2009).

"What to Expect with Menstruation." http://www.kidsgrowth.com/resources/articledetail.cfm?id=772 (accessed 15 June 2009).

Whitlam, J. Collins Dictionary: English–Portuguese, Portugues–Ingles. http://www.credoreference.com.ez.sun.ac.za/vol/501.

Williamson, S., and R. Nowak. "The Truth about Women." New Scientist 159, no. 2145 (1998): 34–35.

Women's Health. "Ageing Down Under." http://www.womhealth.org.au/healthjourney/ageing_down_under.htm (accessed 2 July 2009).

"Women's Health: Body Wisdom for Every Woman." http://www.hudrivctr.org/documents/woman hth.pdf (accessed 24 March 2009).

Woods, N. F. "Exercise, Fitness, and Quality of Life: Implications for Health Promotion for Midlife and Older Women." *The Journal of the North American Menopause Society* 15, no. 4 (2008): 579–80. http://www.ncbi.nlm.nih.gov/pub med/18580540 (accessed 12 March 2012).

Workowski, K. A., and S. M. Berman. "Ectopara-sitic Infections: Sexually Transmitted Diseases Treatment Guidelines." http://www.guideline .gov/summary/summary.aspx?ss=15&doc_id =9687&nbr=5196 (accessed 21 August 2009).

World Health Organization. "Eliminating Female Genital Mutilation: An Interagency Statement." http://www.unfpa.org/webdav/site/global /shared/documents/publications/2008/elimi nating_fgm.pdf (accessed 27 February 2009).

World Health Organization. "Female Genital Muti-lation, Fact Sheet No. 241." http://www.who.int /mediacentre/factsheets/fs241/en (accessed 27 February 2009).

Xiaojia, G., N. Misaki, J. M. Natsuaki, and D. R. Neiderhiser. "Genetic and Environmental Influences on Pubertal Timing: Results from Two National Sibling Studies." *Journal of Re-search on Adolescence* 17, no. 4 (2007): 767–88.

Yates, A. *Sex Without Shame: Encouraging the Child's Healthy Sexual Development.* New York: William Morrow, 1978. http://www.ipce.info /booksreborn/yates/sex/SexWithoutShame .pdf (accessed 1 May 2009).

Yi, H. "Hymen Reconstruction and Plastic Surgery in South Korea." In *The Continuum Complete International Encyclopedia of Sexuality.* Edited by R. T. Francoeur and R. J. Noonan, 944–45. New York: Continuum International Publishing Group, 2004. http://www.kinseyinstitute.org /ccies/kr.php (accessed 17 March 2009).

Youssef, H. "The History of the Condom." *Journal of the Royal Society of Medicine* 86, no. 4 (1993): 226–28.

Zaviacic, M., A. Zaviacicová, J. Komorník, M. Miku-lecký, and I. K. Holomán. "Circatrigintan (30 +/- 5 d) Variations of the Cellular Component of Female Urethral Expulsion Fluid: A Biometrical Study." *International Urology and Nephrology* 16, no. 4 (1984): 311–18.

INDEX

menarche, 48–53

menopause, 10, 79–86

menorrhagia, 124

menstrual pain, 50–51

menstruation: aging and cessation of, 79; days of cycle, average, 46; excessive bleeding during, 124; first (menarche), 48–53; inconvenience of, 28–29; irregular, 125, 138; onset, factors determining, 46, 48–49; pain during, 50–51; pheromones affecting cycle, 22; shame and secrecy of, 49–50; vaginal discharge before, 116

mons pubis (Mound of Venus, mons veneris), 8, 9, 80, 91, 99

muscle strength, 144–145

myths, 76, 142, 144

N

names and nicknames, 4–5, 7, 10, 80, 96, 116

O

obesity, 49

odor, vaginal, 18–26, 44, 121, 138, 149

oral contraceptives, 65–68

oral sex, 64, 129

orgasms, 10, 14–15, 64, 65, 114–115, 147

ovaries, 128

ovulation, 25, 116

P

pain: children and vaginal, 43; endometriosis, 125; G-spot stimulation and, 14–15; gynecological exams, 29; premenstrual and menstrual, 50–51; during sexual intercourse, 72; as STD symptom, 129, 138

pap smears, 133

parasites, 96, 123, 135

pelvic-floor injuries and disorders, 73, 75

pelvic inflammation, 23, 128

pelvic inflammatory disease (PID), 121, 129, 138

pelvic muscles, 10, 13, 65, 81, 82–83

pelvic organ prolapse, 10, 73, 81, 82–83

perfumes, 19, 21, 44, 119, 120

perimenopause, 125

perineal sponge, 5

perineum, 72

personality theories, 96

pH balance, 24–25, 26, 81, 119, 121

pheromones, 21–22, 96

plateau (sexual response stage), 64, 85

playing doctor, 37

Poitiers, Diane de, 144–145

postmenopause, 85–86

pregnancy, 69, 70–73, 75, 116, 118, 124

premenstrual pain, 50

Prince Albert, 93–93

privacy, 34, 36

pseudofolliculitis barbae, 104–108

puberty, 46, 48–53

pubic hair: cutting, shaving and removal of, 96–97, 99, 101, 104–106; menopausal changes and, 80; personality theories and color of, 96; pubescent development of, 46; regrowth and ingrown, 104–108; tribal cleansing rituals, 149

pubococcygeus (PC) muscles, 10